Psychosexual Nursing

Nursing

Robert Irwin BA(Hons), MSc, RGN

*Clinical Nurse Specialist, Sexual Health Team,
Kennet and North Wiltshire Primary Care Trust*

W

WHURR PUBLISHERS

LONDON AND PHILADELPHIA

© 2002 Whurr Publishers
First published 2002 by
Whurr Publishers Ltd
19b Compton Terrace, London N1 2UN, England and
325 Chestnut Street, Philadelphia PA 19106, USA

British Library Cataloguing in Publication Data
A catalogue record for this book is available from the British
Library.

ISBN: 1 86156 341 8

Typeset by HWA Text and Data Management, Tunbridge Wells
Printed and bound in the UK by Athenaeum Press Limited,
Gateshead, Tyne & Wear.

Contents

Acknowledgements

Many thanks to my colleagues Sophie Elkins and Elizabeth Holmes and also to the members of the Bath psychosexual nursing seminar group, who have helped directly and indirectly to develop my ideas about the issues discussed in this book. I also thank Jim McCarthy of Whurr Publishers for inviting me to write this book, and the staff of the Postgraduate Medical Library, Bath and Lyn Norvell of the British Library for their assistance.

This book is dedicated to John Elder whose patience and support made it possible.

Introduction

General practice and specialist sexual health services need to make patients feel that they can discuss problems with their sex lives. Services need to be able to assess patients and refer them on to specialist services when appropriate. (Department of Health, 2001a)

The purpose of this book is to help nurses provide the level of psychosexual care described above. Although this book was written with practitioners who work in primary care and specialist sexual health services specifically in mind, it is hoped that it will be of benefit to practitioners working in all areas of health care. Sexual health is an integral aspect of holistic nursing care and the enhancement and protection of patients' sexual health is dependent upon the sensitivity and skills of practitioners working outside and within the areas of primary care or specialist sexual health services.

The focus of this book is on helping practitioners recognize and respond appropriately to psychosexual anxiety and distress. Recent research suggests that the sexual concerns of patients still go unaddressed and that communication with patients about sexual issues is generally inadequate (Stead et al., 2001). Psychosexual anxiety and distress occur as the consequences of changes or threats to the sexual aspects of an individual's self-concept. Such changes may occur as the consequences of illness, disability, ageing, altered sexual function, relationship difficulties, loss and other psychosocial events. Sexual distress and anxieties that go unrecognized may lead to sexual and interpersonal problems which in turn create further anxiety or distress. As a consequence, a vicious circle of altered sexual self-concept, psychosexual anxiety and distress, and alterations in sexual response and satisfaction, can become quickly established.

It is not the intention of this book to make the reader either an 'expert' in sexual matters, or a psychosexual therapist. The book aims to provide the reader with an outline of an approach to patient care that may help to prevent sexual concerns developing into seemingly intractable sexual or relationship problems that require intensive and protracted specialist intervention. It is recognized that on occasions practitioners will encounter patients with sexual problems who will require referral for specialist help. Consequently, the help that specialist psychosexual services can offer patients and the rationale for referral to such services are discussed.

However, this book does have a number of limitations. The first and possibly most important is that psychosexual nursing skills cannot be acquired by reading a textbook. The acquisition of such skills occurs primarily through experience that is reflected upon and valued (both by the practitioner and others). Inevitably, generalizations have been made in the writing of this text and practitioners should be wary of imposing these on either their patients or themselves. Readers of this book are encouraged to read widely on this subject and recommended reading at the end of each chapter, with a selected biography of further reading at the end of the book, is indicated.

PART I

PRINCIPLES OF PSYCHOSEXUAL NURSING

CHAPTER 1

Psychosexual anxiety and distress

Introduction

Psychosexual anxiety and distress are feelings that arise when an aspect of a person's sexuality is disturbed by a situation or event. Sexuality is a difficult concept to define as it means different things to different people, but generally it refers to something more than just sexual acts or genitalia. Determinants of an individual's sexuality include biological sex, gender identity, sex-role conditioning and sex-role stereotypes (ENB, 1994). Although the term 'sexuality' is often taken to denote something positive about the human condition, it can also serve as conduit for the expression of power, dependency, hatred, manipulation and violence (Savage, 1990). For the purposes of this book, sexuality is viewed as part of an individual's self-concept, shaped throughout life by his or her personality and everyday interactions with others, and expressed as sexual feelings, beliefs and behaviours, through a heterosexual, homosexual, bisexual or transsexual orientation.

When thinking about psychosexual anxiety and distress, it is important to distinguish between those feelings that are a normal, almost expected, reaction to certain events – what Nichols (1993) terms 'functional emotional processes' – and anxiety or distress that leads to psychosexual problems, relationship difficulties or ill-health. It is the latter that is addressed primarily within this text. Psychosexual anxiety and distress may result from:

- Ill-health and/or irreversible anatomical and physiological changes.
- Altered sexual function.

- Sexual dissatisfaction.
- Life events, such as the beginning and ending of relationships, childbirth, growing awareness of aspects of one's sexual identity, ageing, loss and bereavement.

Psychosexual distress may be considered 'problematic' when:

- It impedes recovery from illness or adjustment to chronic health-related conditions.
- It leads or contributes to mental ill-health.
- It alters sexual function in the absence of any underlying physiological cause, or worsens sexual difficulties that are primarily organic in origin.
- It leads to sexual dissatisfaction.
- It contributes to relationship difficulties or breakdown.
- It deters an individual from establishing close, intimate relationships.

In practice, it is sometimes difficult to distinguish between where psychosexual distress that is indicative of 'functional emotional processes' ends and where psychosexual distress and anxiety associated with adverse sequelae actually begins. It is necessary to think about the role and function of such feelings for the individual concerned. When thinking about psychosexual anxiety and distress in relation to ill-health, altered sexual function and interpersonal relationships, it is possible to detect a certain 'circularity'. For example, illness or surgery may lead to psychosexual anxiety that, in turn, alters sexual functioning which results in relationship difficulties and consequently impedes recovery. Asking whether the psychosexual anxiety and distress an individual is experiencing affects adversely his or her general or sexual health, may also help. At this point, it seems an appropriate moment to stop and think about what is meant by the term 'sexual health' and the role of practitioners in general sexual health care.

Defining sexual health

It is generally difficult to find a definition of sexual health that captures the essential components of human sexuality in health and illness and enjoys universal acceptance (Hicken, 1994). In attempting to define sexual health, the World Health Organization (WHO) (WHO, 1986) identifies three key elements:

- A capacity to enjoy and control sexual and reproductive behaviour in accordance with a social and personal ethic.
- Freedom from fear, shame, guilt, false beliefs and other psychological factors inhibiting sexual response and impairing sexual relationships.
- Freedom from organic disorders, diseases and deficiencies that interfere with sexual and reproductive functions.

Savage (1987, p. 25) notes that the above definition of sexual health is concerned with 'reproduction and the erotic aspects of sexuality', thereby neglecting the role of sexual health care in enhancing life and personal relationships. Often, sexual health in nursing practice is equated solely with the prevention of sexually transmitted infections or the provision of contraceptive services.

Cavicchia and Whitehead (1995) raise a number of important questions with regard to the above definition of sexual health, including how does an individual define a 'personal and social ethic'? Given the diversity and ever-changing range of influences and opinions in society, is it ever possible to define an absolute code of behaviour that constitutes a 'social ethic'? Furthermore, how do some individuals cope with changes in their 'personal ethic' that occur over time, or when their opinions and sexual behaviours may be at odds with perceived social norms. Cavicchia and Whitehead (1995) also question how realistic it is to expect individuals to free themselves from fear and shame about sexual identity and practices in a culture that they describe as being essentially 'sex negative'. Finally, given the emphasis placed in the WHO (1986) definition on 'freedom from organic disorders', Cavicchia and Whitehead (1995) ask where this leaves people whose 'organic disorders' cannot be remedied. Does this mean that many people may never attain sexual health? These are important questions and should be kept in mind when thinking about the role of the nurse in psychosexual care as they highlight some common causes of psychosexual anxiety, distress and difficulty:

- Behaviour or feelings that are perceived as deviations from either personal or social 'norms'.
- Internalization of the negativity surrounding sex in our society.
- Assumptions about 'ideals' with regard to sexual expression, gender roles and sexual relationships.

In everyday clinical practice, sexual health may either be a primary or secondary focus of nursing care, depending on the patient's care needs

(RCN, 2000). Savage (1987) observes that the role of the nurse in sexual health care varies according to the nature of a patient's problems, citing three levels of sexual health care in nursing practice. The first of these is described as 'basic sexual health care' and is essentially concerned with the care of the 'non-erotic' aspects of a patient's sexuality, such as self-concept, body image, the management of body boundaries and products, and gender role. Savage (1987) notes that all nurses have a responsibility to provide this level of care. The second level of nursing care is concerned with sexual adjustment, that is helping patients to adjust to sexual changes following ill-health or injury so that patients may re-establish themselves as 'confident individuals who are as sexually active as they want to be' (Savage, 1987, p. 145). The third level of nursing care involves recognizing the ways in which psychosexual problems may be precipitated by ill-health. Savage (1987) suggests that practitioners should have some understanding of what psychosexual treatment involves in order to be able to recognize when referral is appropriate and to discuss with patients what such treatments might involve.

Discussing sexual concerns

A recurring theme of many studies exploring sexual health care and nursing practice, is the wish expressed by many patients that practitioners should initiate any discussion of sexual health, and the reluctance expressed by many practitioners to do so (Waterhouse, 1996). A number of factors may contribute towards this situation.

First, it is important to acknowledge that sexuality is a personal and private part of life for most people, and that privacy needs to be respected by both practitioner and patient (Clifford, 2000a, p. 12). Psychosexual care requires practitioners to remain alert to their patients' expressed and unexpressed needs. The skill required of the practitioner is to demonstrate respect for patients' privacy at the same time as attending to their patients' needs. To do this the practitioner needs to listen with close attention to the feelings that are being expressed, as well as to think about what is *not* being said.

Bor and Watts (1993) note that the context or setting in which conversations with patients take place directly influences the purpose of the discussion, its aims and the content of what can be discussed. Where the patient's presenting problem is primarily of a sexual nature (e.g. urogenital symptoms), most patients anticipate that their sexual relationships will be discussed from the outset. However, both practitioners and patients may experience greater uncertainty and ambivalence about whether or how to discuss sexual problems that are associated with other medical or psychosocial problems (e.g. erectile dysfunction secondary to diabetes) or concern matters not directly related to medical treatment (Bor and Watts, 1993). It is important to note that, even in contexts where discussion of sexual behaviour and sexuality is expected, embarrassment may still lead to the avoidance of certain subjects (Meerabeau, 1999).

Practitioners carry out many physically intimate acts in their everyday clinical practice which might be regarded as sexual if the context or practitioner's motivation were different (Savage, 1987; Lawler, 1991). Savage (1990, p. 25) suggests that 'with this background of intimacy it is difficult to maintain an image of sexual neutrality when nurses invite their patients to give voice to sexual concerns'. This is made more difficult by a 'sexualized' stereotypical image of nurses which leads some patients, relatives and colleagues to target nurses for abuse and sexual harassment. Burnard (2000) notes that when nurses working in the community encounter patients who want to talk about issues relating to sexuality, they need to consider not only if it is appropriate to talk about such matters in another person's home but also whether it is safe to do so. Practitioners may also avoid talking to patients about sexuality when the patient's sexual identity or behaviours pose a direct challenge to aspects of the practitioner's sexuality (Savage, 1987; Guthrie, 1999).

Some practitioners desist from discussing patients' sexual concerns because they fear that addressing this subject merely increases a patient's anxiety. However, this has not been shown to be the case in a number of studies (Waterhouse, 1996). Related to this is the concern that patients may want practitioners to be 'experts' in sexual problems, a role that most practitioners feel they could, and possibly should, not fill (Savage, 1987). Again, no support for this anxiety has been identified in relevant research (Waterhouse, 1996). Other factors identified by some practitioners for not initiating any discussion of patient's sexual concerns is the perception that other nurses do not discuss sex as part of their clinical practice (Kautz et al., 1990), and the lack of time and opportunity to do so (Guthrie, 1999).

Poor training or education in sexuality and sexual health is sometimes cited as a reason for not addressing patients' needs in these areas (RCN, 2000) and this has received considerable attention in certain quarters (Hicken, 1994). There is, however, no conclusive evidence that sexuality education influences clinical practice (Waterhouse, 1996). Some studies have reported notable changes in clinical practice following appropriate education (Matocha and Waterhouse, 1993), whereas others have noted only small changes (Lewis and Bor, 1994) or no change at all (Kautz et al., 1990).

A key question for practitioners considering initiating any discussion of sexual concerns is if a difficulty is identified, what happens next? How do I respond? An approach that is suggested in many nursing texts is the 'PLISSIT' model.

The 'PLISSIT' model of sexual counselling

PLISSIT is an acronym for:

- Permission giving.
- Limited Information.
- Specific Suggestions.
- Intensive Therapy.

This model was developed to describe an approach to individual sex therapy which was primarily behavioural in orientation (Annon, 1976) and which enjoys some popularity as a model for sexual counselling (Butler and Joyce, 1998). In nursing, it serves both as a means of assessing sexual health needs (McNall, 2000; RCN, 2000) and as a model for sexual counselling and teaching within clinical practice (Waterhouse, 1996; Muir, 2000; White, 2001). As a model for sexual counselling within nursing practice it is essentially a form of 'advisory counselling' in that much of the communication is from practitioner to patient (Nichols, 1993). Advisory, as opposed to personal, counselling tends to be concerned with giving information and advice, and is generally directive in nature (Nichols, 1993, p. 143).

'Permission giving', the first level of the PLISSIT approach, involves 'conveying to the patient that sexuality is a suitable subject for discussion and providing assurance that concerns and practices are normal' (Waterhouse, 1996). Waterhouse (1996) suggests that all nurses should be able to function at this level and notes that most nurses can also intervene at the next level by providing 'limited information'. This involves providing limited factual information which is relevant to the patient's primary health concerns or problem. Limited information may also involve addressing any myths or misconceptions the patient may have. Making 'specific suggestions' to help patients who are experiencing particular sexual difficulties is deemed to be beyond the knowledge and skills of most practitioners (Waterhouse, 1996). This level of intervention is generally provided by nurses who have completed training at a 'specialist practitioner level' (RCN, 2000; White, 2001). Patients with long-standing sexual problems or severely stressed relationships may require 'intensive therapy' and this should only be undertaken by practitioners who have completed specialist training in, for example, psychosexual therapy or relationship counselling (Waterhouse, 1996; RCN, 2000; White, 2001). Accordingly, most practitioners would be expected to refer patients who require help at this level.

One of the tenets of this approach is the validation of patient's sexuality and sexual expression. Webb (1985) suggests that practitioners who understand the diversity of human sexual expression:

> can validate the "normality" and acceptability of any sexual practice which is freely consented to and pleasurable to participants, and help lift the unnecessary burdens of guilt which can interfere with sexual enjoyment. (Webb, 1985, p. 155)

However, as Savage (1987) observes, many nurses, like much of the general population, retain certain 'limiting assumptions' about human sexuality. The first of these is the 'heterosexual assumption'. Linked closely to this is the 'intercourse assumption' that equates 'sex' with penile–vaginal penetration, thereby ignoring other forms of sexual expression. The final assumption Savage (1987) notes is to do with age, specifically the denial of sexuality in both children and the elderly. It would seem that for many nurses even providing care at the first level of the PLISSIT model for certain patients might prove problematic.

The second and third levels of the PLISSIT model – 'limited information' and 'specific suggestions' – are interventions that may help prevent the development of psychosexual anxiety and distress in patients undergoing changes in health or treatment, and correspond to the notion of 'informational and educational care' described by Nichols (1993). As with any form of informational care:

> the work of assessing a person's knowledge and expectations must be emphasized to the same degree as actually giving information – that is prior to and after the communication of significant information, it becomes standard practice to check what a person knows, how accurate and complete this is, and what expectations they generate from the material (Nichols, 1993, p. 79)

The PLISSIT approach to sexual counselling may benefit patients who are experiencing sexual difficulties that are the consequence of problems such as ignorance, misunderstanding or some degree of unjustified guilt or anxiety (Bancroft, 1989). Bancroft (1989) notes that although many professionals are able to offer this type of 'simple counselling', it does have certain requirements, the importance of which should not be underestimated. Chief among these are that practitioners feel relaxed and comfortable with sexual issues, have sufficient knowledge to be confidently informative and are skilled at recognizing communication difficulties and teaching basic communication skills.

The notion of 'expertise' permeates the PLISSIT approach as it is applied to nursing care. One of the advantages of this model is that it allows practitioners to intervene at a level commensurate with their knowledge and skills as well as their level of personal comfort. This perceived strength of the PLISSIT model may also be its primary weakness in terms of psychosexual care. First, the focus of the PLISSIT approach is on practitioner-directed 'problem-solving'. Implicit in this is the notion that the solutions to a patient's difficulties lie outside the patient (in the form of the practitioner's knowledge or skills), whereas one of the major premises of psychosexual care is recognizing 'that patients have the information within themselves that can enable them to resolve their sexual problems in a way that will suit them best' (Wakley, 1998, p. 149). Although the PLISSIT model places emphasis on 'knowing' and 'doing', little attention is given to the practitioner's 'professional use of the self' in this process, which is an essential aspect of what has been termed 'psychosexual awareness' (Clifford, 1998b; Clifford, 2000a). In psychosexual care, like emotional care in general, the process is as important as the content. Indeed, the PLISSIT model, like the 'nursing process' (see Fabricius, 1991), rather than reducing the depersonalization and distance in the nurse–patient relationship, may actually act as a means of defence against awareness in practitioners, of a patient's emotional distress.

The presentation of psychosexual problems

The presentation of psychosexual distress is often indirect or covert. Many patients with psychosexual problems seldom come straight to the point when attempting to disclose their difficulties, as they often fear looking ignorant because of using the wrong words, causing offence by being too explicit or have no way of conceptualizing what is wrong (Selby, 1989, 2000). Consequently, any mention of a sexual difficulty is often extremely tentative and couched in euphemism (Ramage, 1998).

Some patients may feel ashamed or even humiliated at having to ask for help with something that they think is private and that they should be able to cope with themselves (Tomlinson, 1998). Rogers (1989, p. 26) observes that 'it is often quite impossible for embarrassed people to confront another person openly and straightforwardly with their problems', and consequently, people waiting to communicate something of embarrassment to themselves, often create difficulties around getting or attending appointments. Such behaviour can leave health professionals, who may have gone to some considerable trouble to accommodate a patient, feeling manipulated, undervalued and annoyed. This, in turn, may militate against a sympathetic reception for the patient when he or she eventually does attend.

Emotional pain or conflict can be converted into physical pain and sometimes another symptom or complaint, such as depression or insomnia, or unexplained genital symptoms may indicate the presence of psychosexual problem (Hawton, 1985; Ramage, 1998; Smith, 2001). Persisting concerns about having a sexually transmitted infection or frequent visits to discuss methods of contraception may all be ways of trying to communicate psychosexual distress (Rogers, 1989; Christopher, 1996). Indeed, certain clinical areas, such as family planning and genitourinary medicine, may be perceived as more 'legitimate' arenas for bringing and possibly unpacking the 'emotional baggage of sex gone wrong' (Crowley, 1997). On occasions, complaints about partners may indicate sexual fears, anxieties and difficulties on the part of a patient. The tendency for some patients to perceive the sole responsibility for a sexual difficulty as residing in their partners should be treated with caution.

Some patients may persistently attend with seemingly minor or non-specific complaints. Often, this is a form of 'testing out' of the health professional by patients and such behaviour may continue until the patient feels secure enough with a practitioner to mention what is truly troubling him or her without fear of being judged, ridiculed or rejected. This may explain why some patients only begin to address what is truly concerning them as a consultation is ending – the 'hand on the door' disclosure – as it feels safer to disclose at the end of the consultation, when very little time is left, than at the beginning. In such a situation patients know that their distress is 'contained' as there is insufficient time for the problem to be discussed 'in depth', and if the problem is dismissed by the practitioner they do not need to come back. Although such consultation behaviour may be frustrating for the practitioner, these disclosures do need to be acknowledged and explored briefly before the patient can be asked to come back when there is more time. Ignoring what the patient has said or seeking to dismiss the significance of the patient's disclosure with platitudes or hasty reassurance may mean the patient either never attends again or never seeks to bring up the problem again and the opportunity to help may have been lost for ever.

Psychosexual care requires a psychosomatic approach to patient care. This means recognizing that the mind and the body are entwined to such an extent that changes in one may cause changes in the other (Clifford, 2000a). Hence, when thoughts and feelings are disturbed, bodily functions are also liable to be disturbed and, conversely, changes in the body bring about changes in the mind. Sexual function provides a prime example of such a psychosomatic process (*see* Bancroft, 1989, pp 373–405). Psychosexual anxiety and distress may find expression in disturbed interpersonal relationships, somatically, in the form of bodily symptoms, or, most commonly, as a combination of both these phenomena. The challenge for practitioners is to become aware of their patients' psychosexual anxiety and distress and to respond effectively to these feelings.

Psychosexual awareness

Clifford (2000a, p. 20) defines psychosexual awareness as 'the integration into one's practice of the facts of human sexuality and its vulnerability'. Psychosexual awareness is dependent on the 'professional use of the self', that is, the practitioner's use of their own individuality whilst relating to the patient in a professional way. The focus of this approach to psychosexual care is how practitioners manage the boundary between personal involvement and professional detachment, particularly when faced with people who are in distress (Clifford, 2000a).

Like the PLISSIT approach, there is emphasis placed on facilitating a relationship between nurse and patient which enables any psychosexual difficulties to be acknowledged and shared. The analogy for this process in many of the texts written about psychosexual awareness is that of 'building a bridge for the patient to cross in safety' (Clifford, 1998b). Clifford (1998b) notes that the image of a bridge conveys that whilst an offer is being made by the practitioner to attend to the patient's feelings, there is no obligation for the patient to accept such an offer, thus preserving the patient's right to privacy (Clifford, 2000a). Clifford (2000a, p. 31) observes that such 'bridge building' has certain requirements, including the confidence to be available to and respond with closeness to another, the confidence to emerge from 'behind the defence of knowledge' and the confidence to take the risk of listening without the certainty of answers.

A number of assumptions underpin the concept of psychosexual awareness. The first is that the experience of physical or psychological distress stimulates in most people a similar need to find someone else to share and hold that pain. A second, related assumption is that psychosexual difficulties are the consequence of protective barriers erected by patients in the face of pain, anxiety or distress. The third assumption of this approach to psychosexual care is that given the appropriate therapeutic space patients can become aware of their own pain and generate their own resolution to their psychosexual difficulties.

Penman (1998) suggests that the two traditional models of nurse–patient relationship, namely the 'expert nurse–vulnerable patient' and 'maternal (paternal) nurse–dependent patient' militate against the creation of a therapeutic space between practitioner and patient, though for different reasons. In the 'expert nurse–vulnerable patient' paradigm there is perceived to be too much distance between the patient and nurse. The practitioner appears confident but distant, resorts to speaking from a theoretical base and expects to provide the solution for the patient's difficulties. Consequently, the patient is required to minimize his or her distress, is not called upon to offer an understanding of his or her own difficulties and is expected to leave responsibility to the 'expert' to solve the problem. In the 'maternal (paternal) nurse–dependent patient' paradigm, the patient's own potential for discovering solutions to his or her psychosexual difficulties is smothered by 'the nurse's need to find or offer comfort in the form of professional theories, personal ideas and assumptions' (Penman, 1998, p. 49). Such actions on the part of practitioners may lead to the patient temporarily feeling better, but no significant change occurs in the underlying psychosexual problem as the patient has been denied the opportunity to 'hear' his or her own anxiety or distress. Penman (1998) indicates that therapeutic space for the patient to discover the relationship between his or her own emotions and somatic symptoms occurs when the practitioner allows him- or herself not to know, or presume to know the answers, but observes all the that the patient brings to the consultation. 'Freed' by the 'unknowing' of the nurse, the patient is able to become aware of his or her own pain, anxiety and distress and the consequent protective barriers that cause psychosexual difficulties.

A number of factors may facilitate or impede the ability of practitioners to 'hear' a patient's psychosexual distress and create a therapeutic space in which this can be worked with. The provision of intimate acts of care, such as taking a cervical smear or urogenital swabs, no matter how impeccably carried out, potentially disturb patients' sense of their own private space (Nicolson, 1998) and may trigger reactions indicative of psychosexual anxiety or distress (Selby, 1989). The study of the interaction in the nurse–patient relationship can also generate insight into the patient's problem. Selby (1989) notes that this requires the 'nurse to be able, not only to listen and feel with the patient, but also to be able to think about what is happening in the "here and now" '. The practitioner's own emotional response to the patient may parallel how the patient is feeling, or may indicate how the patient is experienced by others such as his or her partner(s). It is suggested that the skills required for this way of working with patients may be developed in Balint-style psychosexual seminar training groups (Clifford, 1998a; Penman, 1998; Wells, 2000).

During Balint-style psychosexual training seminars, practitioners are invited to describe encounters with patients, especially those that have left them feeling uneasy or dissatisfied with the response they have offered. The purpose of the group is to attend carefully to the practitioner's description of the encounter and explore the nature of the interaction between practitioner and patient. This, in turn, may generate awareness in the practitioner of some of the emotions and dynamics that characterized the encounter with the patient. Such groups also provide an environment in which to explore the types of professional behaviours that serve as defences when the 'here and now' of the nurse–patient relationship becomes too uncomfortable or threatening. Some defences are necessary to ensure that practitioners are able to function in order to benefit patients, whereas others interrupt the therapeutic function of the nurse. Examples of such defences include choosing not to 'hear' the patient's pain and distress, 'ritualization' (the use of techniques and interventions about which the practitioner has no real knowledge or experience), deferring patients who wish to discuss their feelings until a 'more appropriate' time or situation arises, and inappropriate referral (Selby, 1989). Labelling patients may also be a way of avoiding having to think about their pain and distress.

In contrast to the 'behaviourist' origins of the PLISSIT approach, psychosexual awareness has developed from a psychodynamic tradition (*see* Barnes et al., 1998; Wells, 2000). There is a greater emphasis in psychosexual awareness on 'being', compared with the 'knowing' and 'doing', in the nurse–patient relationship. To some patients, who perhaps perceive health practitioners as 'experts' who will generate instant solutions to their psychosexual problems, this approach may rankle. Equally, for many practitioners remaining 'unknowing' when faced with a distressed patient requires them to contain the impetus to 'do something' conferred upon them by their professional socialization.

Key points of Chapter 1

- Psychosexual care is concerned with recognizing and responding appropriately to psychosexual anxiety and distress.
- Psychosexual anxiety and distress may be both an antecedent and a consequence of ill-health, altered sexual function or the stress associated with certain life events.
- It is important, but sometimes very difficult, to distinguish between psychosexual distress that is a normal response to certain events and psychosexual distress that leads to psychosexual problems and relationship difficulties.
- Psychosexual anxiety and distress may find expression in disturbed interpersonal relationships, somatically in the form of bodily symptoms, or as a combination of both these phenomena. Consequently, a psychosomatic approach is required to patient care.
- The presentation of psychosexual difficulties is often indirect or covert. Psychosexual distress may become apparent during the provision of physical care that is intimate in nature or through an awareness of the emotions present in the 'here and now' of the nurse–patient relationship.
- There is evidence from a number of studies which suggests that many patients would prefer practitioners to initiate any discussion of sexual concerns, but many practitioners are reluctant to do so.
- The challenge for practitioners with regard to psychosexual care is to develop an approach to patient care that both acknowledges and responds to patients' needs, and at the same time demonstrates respect for the patient's privacy.
- In psychosexual care, as in emotional care in general, the process is as important as the content.
- A central premise of working with patients with psychosexual problems is that patients have within themselves the information that can enable them to resolve their difficulties in a way that will suit them best.
- The challenge for practitioners is to create a therapeutic space within the nurse–patient relationship, which is sufficient to enable patients to become aware of their own feelings and how these relate to their psychosexual difficulties. This requires the practitioner to remain 'unknowing' in the face of distress.

- The development in practitioners of the skills required for 'psychosexual awareness' may help with this process of care.

Key reading

Penman, J. (1998) Action research in the care of patients with sexual anxieties. *Nursing Standard* **13**, 13–15, 47–50.

White, I. (2001) Facilitating sexual expression: challenges for contemporary practice. In: Heath, H., White, I. (eds). *The Challenge of Sexuality in Health Care*. Oxford: Blackwell Science.

CHAPTER 2

Professional issues in psychosexual care

Introduction

The nurse–patient relationship is an example of a 'fiduciary relationship'. Fiduciary relationships are relationships in which one person (in this case the practitioner) accepts the trust and confidence of another to act in the other's best interest. The need for the patient to trust a nurse places the nurse in a position of power within that relationship.

The safety of patients within the nurse–patient relationship is dependent in part on how the practitioner exercises this power. This is determined by the practitioner's response to his or her professional, contractual and legal obligations, and by his or her ethical reasoning (RCN, 2000; Wilson, 2000). 'Ethics' refers to the moral philosophy and reasoning adopted by an individual to justify his or her actions. An approach to moral reasoning often used in health care settings is that devised by Beauchamp and Childress (1989). Beauchamp and Childress (1989) describe four moral principles that they suggest are binding unless in a given situation a certain principle assumes more significance and overrides the others. These principles are: respect for autonomy; beneficence; non-maleficence; and justice. The principle of respect for autonomy is founded on two values: the freedom of an individual to make her or his own choices, and the freedom to decide their own actions. This concept of free choice is not unlimited as it is bounded axiomatically by respect for the autonomy of others. Beneficence refers to caring for and working to promote the greatest good for others, whereas non-maleficence – the principle of 'doing no harm' – values the responsible use of power and ability. The principle of justice refers the valuing of fairness and the equal distribution of costs and benefits.

In terms of psychosexual care there are two overarching and related requirements to ensure the safety of patients, namely, establishing and maintaining appropriate professional boundaries within the nurse–patient relationship and ensuring no act or omission on the part of the practitioner is detrimental to the patient's well-being.

Boundaries

What are boundaries and what purpose do they serve in the nurse–patient relationship? The United Kingdom Central Council for Nursing, Midwifery and Health Visiting (UKCC) (UKCC, 1999, p. 5) suggests that 'boundaries define the limits of behaviour which allow a client and a practitioner to engage safely in a therapeutic caring relationship'. Boundaries are particularly important in nursing care as they enable nurses to perform acts, for example touching patients when carrying out intimate body care or asking very personal questions, that would in other social contexts be deemed unacceptable. Given the position of power which the practitioner enjoys in the nurse–patient relationship, it remains the practitioner's responsibility to maintain professional boundaries within the relationship at all times (UKCC, 1999).

As discussed in Chapter 1, the presentation of psychosexual difficulties may often be indirect or covert, reflecting the embarrassment and difficulty many patients have with disclosing such problems (Rogers, 1989). The disclosure of sensitive and private information places patients in an increasingly vulnerable position and a number of professional behaviours serve to ensure patient safety. These include:

- Maintaining confidentiality.
- Recognizing and respecting the uniqueness and dignity of each patient.
- Avoiding any abuse of the privileged relationship with patients.

Confidentiality

To provide another person with private and personal information about oneself is a significant act of trust. Disclosure in psychosexual care may mean patients sharing information about their thoughts, feelings and behaviour that they may not have previously acknowledged to themselves, let alone to others. The boundary of confidentiality helps to create a therapeutic space in which a patient may acknowledge thoughts, feelings and acts that may feel unacceptable, disturbing or dangerous to him or her. This is necessary if a patient is to discover the unique connections between what he or she is feeling and the somatic and sexual symptoms he or she may be experiencing. In this sense, confidentiality helps to provide some form of containment for the patient in that he or she can acknowledge and explore distressing and disturbing thoughts and feelings in a situation where there is sense of safety generated by the fact that such information will not be shared elsewhere. However, this can only ever be partial containment, as the notion of confidentiality is not absolute in health care settings. According to clause 10 of the *Code of Professional Conduct* (UKCC, 1992), practitioners are required to:

> protect all confidential information concerning patients and clients obtained in the course of professional practice and make disclosures only with consent, where required by the order of a court or where you can justify disclosure in the wider public interest;
> (UKCC, 1992)

McHale (1998) notes that the extent of this obligation is defined by guidance issued by the UKCC (1996a), the practitioner's contract of employment and the law, in that where information has been disclosed in breach of this obligation of confidence, legal proceedings may follow. In addition to this general obligation of confidentiality, certain specific obligations of confidentiality have been imposed on practitioners by statute. Section 33 of the Human Fertilisation and Embryology Act, 1990, places a statutory ban upon the disclosure of information about gamete donors and patients receiving treatment under the Act. Unauthorized disclosure of such information by health care professionals and others (save under certain exceptions) is a criminal offence. The National Health Service Venereal Disease Regulations (1974) require that health authorities should ensure that information relating to people being treated for sexually transmitted diseases should not be disclosed, except where this is for the purpose of communicating the information to a doctor caring for the patient, or to a person working under the direction of that doctor to treat that condition or to prevent its spread.

Jenkins (1999) observes that within health care settings, and unlike many other therapeutic settings, a 'structural' model of confidentiality generally operates which includes reference to crucial aspects, such as risk assessment and sharing information within a multi-disciplinary team. This reflects the fact that it is impracticable to obtain the consent of a patient every time there is a need to share information with other health professionals involved in the care of that patient. The UKCC (1996a) acknowledges this, but states that it is important that patients understand that some information may be made available to others involved in the delivery of their care and that patients must know with whom that information will be shared.

As the *Code of Professional Conduct* (UKCC, 1992) indicates, there are exceptional circumstances in which practitioners may be required to disclose information without the patient's consent. Such situations include when required to do so by law or by order of a court, or when after careful consideration disclosure is deemed to be necessary in the wider public interest. The UKCC (1996a, p. 27) defines the 'wider public interest' as:

> the interests of an individual, or groups of individuals or of society as a whole, and would, for example, cover matters such as serious crime, child abuse, drug trafficking or other activities which place others at serious risk.'

This has particular pertinence for the practice of psychosexual care as certain sexual acts are serious criminal offences (e.g. child sex abuse or rape) and in certain circumstances some sexual activities might be deemed to place others at 'serious risk'. A number of factors may influence the decision to disclose information in the wider public interest. From an ethical point of view, practitioners considering breaching their obligation of confidentiality in the wider public interest have to balance the principle of non-maleficence towards others against that of respecting the patient's autonomy. Grubin (1999) suggests that in attempting to resolve dilemmas about protecting potential victims from harm, it is important to disentangle personal from professional views. He notes that although as an ordinary member of society one is entitled to have a 'low threshold' in relation to disclosing information relevant to the safety of other individuals, the professional, as opposed to the citizen, must consider a number of factors, including the extent to which risk can be quantified, whether risk really will be reduced by disclosure and 'whether the short-term gain achieved by disclosure will be at the expense of an increase in risk in the long term, which might occur if the therapeutic relationship is brought to an end by the disclosure, thus negating any possibility of a future reduction in risk though treatment or monitoring' (Grubin, 1999, pp 281–282).

Grubin (1999, p. 282) suggests that the following principles, if adopted, may be applied to ethical dilemmas associated with 'sexually dangerous' individuals. In order for a breach of confidentiality to be justified as being in the wider public interest, it must be shown that:

- The risk is 'real, immediate and serious'.

- The risk will be reduced by disclosure.
- Disclosure is no more than that required to reduce risk.
- Any damage to the public interest in relation to broken confidentiality is outweighed by the public interest of reducing risk.

Before making any decision about whether to release information without a patient's permission, practitioners should always discuss matters fully with other professional colleagues and, if appropriate, consult the UKCC or a membership organization. Once a decision has been made, it (with the reasons for it) and any concomitant actions should be documented either in the appropriate record or as a special note kept in a separate file. In terms of maintaining patient safety, practitioners need to ensure that from the outset patients are aware that confidentiality is not an absolute principle. Patients need to be informed that in certain circumstances information may be shared on a 'need to know basis' with other colleagues involved in their care. It should also be pointed out that there are certain exceptional circumstances, including when it is deemed to be in the wider public interest, when a practitioner may be obliged to disclose certain information without the patient's consent.

Recognizing and respecting the uniqueness and dignity of the individual

This is an obligation stated in clause 7 of the *Code of Professional Conduct* (UKCC, 1992) and its importance has been reiterated in *Practitioner–client Relationships and the Prevention of Abuse* (UKCC, 1999). Clause 7 of the *Code of Professional Conduct* (UKCC, 1992) also requires practitioners to respond to patients' need for care 'irrespective of their ethnic origin, religious beliefs, personal attributes, the nature of their health problem or any other factors'. The obligations set out in clause 7 reflect the growing shift towards an holistic and individualized approach to patient care. Hayter (1996) observes that the concept of holistic care and the increasing importance placed on the relationship between nurse and patient have created a range of difficulties that have until recently received little attention. Some of these difficulties relate to the particular challenges which sexuality and sexual health present to the personal morality and values of some practitioners.

Given Webb's (1985) assertion that:

> Sexuality involves the totality of being a person and therefore nurses and patients are only given their full respect as people when nursing care has firm foundations in a

truly holistic approach incorporating sexuality as a vital aspect of humanity (Webb, 1985, p. 147)

it is impossible to recognize and respect the uniqueness and dignity of an individual without reference to his or her sexuality. Some authors suggest that there is a general proclivity, certainly during the process of making a nursing assessment, for practitioners to view patients as 'asexual'. The denial of a patient's sexuality may extend beyond a casual omission to fill in the 'sexuality' section on the nursing assessment document (Gamlin, 1999) to an active, but erroneous, construction of certain patients as being without sexuality or sexual health needs. Commonly, this occurs with patients belonging to the following groups:

- People with learning disabilities.
- People with mental health problems.
- Children.
- The elderly.
- People with physical or sensory disabilities.

Some of the most frequently cited examples of disregard for the uniqueness and dignity of individual patients relate to the 'care' of patients who are gay, lesbian or bisexual. Heterosexism (the belief in the superiority or universality of heterosexual relationships) and homophobia (the fear or hatred of same-sex attraction and relationships) at both an individual and institutional level militate against patients who are gay or lesbian receiving high-quality care in certain circumstances (RCN, 1994). The findings of part of a recent interview study of the experiences of nursing care of lesbians and gay men generated the following themes (with regard to the experiences of lesbian interviewees):

- Concern that disclosure would lead to feelings of vulnerability and powerlessness;
- Heterosexism makes disclosure difficult and affects the accuracy of treatment and diagnosis. This in turn restricts access to appropriate care, advice and support;
- Homophobic reactions to disclosure, including physical, verbal, non-verbal and sexual abuse;
- Ignorance among professionals about the health needs, lives and concerns of lesbian women. (Platzer and James, 2000, p. 195)

These themes reflect the findings of other studies that indicate that the disclosure of sexual orientation has lead to the experience of neglect, loss of dignity and inadequate health care provision for some patients. A sense of avoidance, abandonment and distancing (on the part of nursing staff) has been reported by patients in some studies, as has the converse situation, whereby gay men and lesbians have been subjected to almost voyeuristic attention (RCN, 1994; Taylor and Robertson, 1994; Morrisey and Rivers, 1998; Albarran and Salmon, 2000). Caulfield and Platzer (1998) also note the tendency of some practitioners to disregard the requests of patients who have wanted their same-sex partner recognized and respected as their next of kin.

Christopher (1996) observes that psychosexual difficulties are a characteristic of every society, but it is whether and how the problems present and what is expected from treatment that may vary considerably between members of differing ethnic or cultural groups (*see also* d'Ardenne, 1988; Bhui, 1998). Although greater awareness and knowledge of the differences that exist between different cultural, ethnic and religious communities may facilitate psychosexual care, Pollen (2001), writing on 'cultural aspects of sexual difficulties' suggests that this can lead to the categorization of patients in what she terms 'essentialist terms', that is, 'describing people as if they had a fixed essence determined strongly by the category in question (ethnicity, genes, gender, social class, nationality, culture)' (Pollen, 2001, p. 4). Pollen (2001) suggests that such essentialism may distract practitioners from the relationship that exists between them and their patients and may actually steer practitioners towards stereotyping and prejudice. Pollen (2001) advocates remaining as grounded as possible in the 'here and now' practitioner–patient relationship and moving cautiously outwards from this point to look for aspects of the relationship which appear to have become involved with cultural issues. She suggests that 'the power of empathetically gained subjective knowledge' neutralizes the tendency to bias and prejudice that is often present in so-called 'objective observation', and also advocates examining practitioner–patient relationships which appear to have become 'culturalized' (in the same way that professional relationships may be 'sexualized') rather than creating a 'mental database of cultural traits and imposing this from the top down, making an essentialist or stereotyped typology of patients' (Pollen, 2001, p. 5).

However, there remain a number of significant issues for practitioners to consider with regard to 'cross-cultural' psychosexual care. There is, for example, a very strong proscription within certain cultures with regard to when, and with whom, sexual matters may be discussed. Language difficulties may necessitate the use of translators. Using informal translators (such as partners, other family members) is generally not recommended, but professional interpreters are often difficult to access. It is important to remember that the presence of a 'third party', even if it is a 'professional interpreter', may alter the dynamics of the nurse–patient relationship. Although words may be translated literally, the meaning conveyed in the choice of particular words, their significance to the speaker and the way they are spoken, may be lost in translation.

Making the assumption that someone who is perceived to be from a certain cultural or ethnic group automatically subscribes unswervingly to a certain 'dominant' value or belief system associated with that group is an example of 'essentialist' thinking. Christopher (1996) observes that many individuals may well be at a transitional stage between their culture of origin and that of their place of birth and residence. She suggests that this may lead to 'inter-generational conflict between those (usually the old) who wish to preserve their culture and those (usually the young) who wish to abandon it wholesale or partially' (Christopher, 1996, p. 25). Whilst the shift in relation to cultural norms and expectations may not always be in the direction indicated by Christopher (1996), Christopher's (1996) observations do serve as a reminder that psychosexual difficulties may be the consequence of conflicts between values or beliefs about sexuality and sexual relationships that are either intra-personal (within oneself) or inter-personal (between individuals). Pollen (2001, p. 6) makes the important observation that 'there is nothing fixed about the relationship between any particular cultural precept and how it affects the sexual life of individuals in practice'. Furthermore, just as 'negative' stereotyping – where practitioners hold rigid and therefore ultimately oppressive views about the sexuality and sexual behaviour of patients from differing races or cultures – interferes with psychosexual care, so can assuming that a patient of the same ethnic or cultural background shares the same beliefs, attitudes, perceptions and experiences as oneself.

Stereotyping and psychosexual care

Stereotypes are generalized beliefs about the characteristics of members of an identifiable group – these beliefs may be positive or negative. When stereotyping interferes with the accurate perception of the characteristics of a particular individual it may have adverse effects on the nurse–patient relationship. A further difficulty with stereotypes is that they are often resistant to change because they create a sense of solidarity with others who hold them. There are a number of social forces that create and maintain negative stereotypes of individuals from certain groups and these forces may influence practitioners and patients alike. Stereotyping may apply to people of differing physical and intellectual abilities, gender, sexual orientation, ethnicity, social class or religious conviction. A further difficulty with stereotypes is that they are often automatically triggered when people with different characteristics or attributes are encountered. This has implications in terms of providing psychosexual care.

Negative stereotyping of patients may lead practitioners to either avoid or distance themselves from certain patients. Forms of distancing include ensuring that nurse–patient interaction remains essentially what Morse (1991, p. 458) terms as a 'clinical relationship', that is, employing certain interactional strategies to ensure conversations with certain patients are limited to nursing tasks such as drug therapy or discharge arrangements. Too great a distance between practitioner and patient often results in the patient's sexuality and sexual health needs remaining unacknowledged.

Caring for a patient with attributes that are viewed negatively by a practitioner may create a sense of dissonance for that practitioner (Johnson and Webb, 1995; Hayter, 1996). 'Dissonance' refers to the psychological discomfort produced by attitudes that are inconsistent with behaviour, which in turn creates pressure to change those attitudes. Guthrie (1999) notes that such dissonance occurred for some of the respondents in her study in relation to caring for patients who were gay. She observes that whilst respondents recognized they were bound by their professional code of conduct to care for gay patients they felt unable to do so because of their own beliefs and attitudes. Guthrie (1999) suggests one of the ways these practitioners responded to this dissonance was to avoid talking to gay patients about their sexuality. Often it is the non-verbal cues indicating nurses' dislike or disapproval that patients pick up on. Emotional distancing on the part of the practitioner may be evident to patients in the practitioner's tone of voice, facial expression and use of touch (Hayter, 1996). Conversely, some patients may anticipate prejudice from practitioners and, even when this is not present, this may still lead to patients avoiding any reference to their sexual identity, behaviour or concerns. In each of these situations there is insufficient safety in the nurse–patient relationship for the patient to reveal his or her anxieties.

Recognition of the patient's feelings through resonance in one's own is a key psychosexual nursing skill (Clifford, 2000a, 2000b), that is explored further in Chapter 3 of this book. Clifford (2000a) suggests that some of the feelings practitioners may experience in response to particular patients are acceptable, whereas others are considered difficult. Certain feelings are deemed 'unacceptable' and are hard for practitioners (and patients) to recognize and accept. Such unacceptable feelings include fear, dislike, contempt, anger and disgust. However, such feelings may also be the consequence of negative stereotyping, and in encounters with patients whom practitioners stereotype, the 'unacceptable' feelings experienced may be a response to a stereotype rather than the feelings that a patient as an individual finds difficult to acknowledge or accept. Hayter (1996) asserts that clinical supervision, if properly set up, can help practitioners to limit the impact of preconceptions about their patients, by acknowledging attitudes and being able to ventilate feelings and discuss methods of coping. He does, however, acknowledge that although reflective practice and clinical supervision may help they are not a panacea for all difficulties in the caring relationship that are the consequence of practitioners' attitudes.

Avoiding any abuse of the health professional's privileged relationship with patients

This is the requirement of clause 9 of the UKCC (1992) *Code of Conduct* and includes avoiding any abuse of the privileged access that a practitioner might have to the patient's person, property, residence or workplace. Green (1999) notes that the nature of the privileged relationship practitioners have with their patients has a number of different aspects, including intimate knowledge of the patient (often gained by being present when patients are at their most vulnerable, for example when they are in pain, anxious, confused or afraid) and influence on patients. This influence, which often derives from the perceived 'expertise' of practitioners or the dependency that some patients have on practitioners for their basic needs to be met, can have powerful psychological effects on both patient and practitioner. Green (1999) suggests that the strongest influence practitioners may exert over patients occurs when practitioners act as counsellors. In such circumstances, patients who are often already vulnerable become more so because of the self-expression involved. Therefore, when practitioners and patients engage in close therapeutic relationships, the potential and opportunity for the relationship to develop in an improper manner increase (UKCC, 1999).

Because psychosexual care requires the 'professional use of the self' practitioners should be wary of entering into a 'dual relationship' with a patient. Dual relationships occur when the practitioner either serves two professional roles for a patient or where the professional relationship includes certain personal elements. Dual relationships may occur successively as well as concurrently (Plaut, 1997). Plaut (1997) observes that dual relationships become problematic:

(a) when the dual aspect of the relationship compromises professional effectiveness;
(b) when the patient becomes concerned about or harmed by factors related to the dual features of the relationship; and
(c) when observers of the relationship find that the dual nature of the relationship compromises the effectiveness of the professional environment. (Plaut, 1997, p. 84)

The UKCC states that the therapeutic caring relationship between practitioner and patient must focus solely on the health care needs of patients. Such relationships are not established to build personal and social contacts for practitioners. Furthermore, 'moving the focus of care from meeting the client's needs towards meeting the practitioner's own needs is an unacceptable abuse of power' (UKCC, 1999, p. 5). Selby (1989) observes that because of the close relationship between practitioners and some of their patients there is a temptation to allow the relationship to develop into friendship. She notes that 'personal relationships and loyalties always get in the way of psychosexual work and should not be allowed to develop' (Selby, 1989, p. 141).

Sexual attraction

It is quite normal that on occasions practitioners may have strong feelings towards a patient and vice versa (Savage, 1987; Plaut, 1997, UKCC, 1999). Such feelings are neither abnormal nor wrong, but would compromise the relationship if the practitioner acted upon them improperly. It is important to recognize that working on psychosexual issues may increase the risk of inappropriate behaviour entering the nurse–patient relationship. Psychosexual care may sometimes involve listening to a patient disclose sexually explicit information which has a highly erotic content. On such occasions practitioners may sometimes find that they become sexually aroused. This increases the risk of inappropriate acts occurring, such as asking questions about the patient's sex life which are salacious in origin, extending unduly the duration of a particular consultation, arranging to meet the patient outside the clinical setting or touching the patient inappropriately. Even when feelings of sexual attraction are not acted upon, they still may affect patient care adversely. Savage (1987) suggests that nurses employ two types of coping strategies when they find themselves sexually attracted to a patient. Practitioners either avoid the patient as far as possible, developing an 'offhand' manner with him or her, or become closely involved with the patient and reluctant to allow him or her space to regain independence. Both of these coping strategies militate against the provision of psychosexual care and indicate once again the need for all practitioners to have access to high-quality clinical supervision.

Sexual abuse

There are certain circumstances in which a sexual relationship with a patient would also be a criminal act. Under Section 128 of the Mental Health Act (1959), any male member of staff in a psychiatric hospital or nursing home who has sexual intercourse with a female patient of the same institution commits an offence. The Sexual Offences (Amendment) Act (2000) makes it an offence to have sexual intercourse (whether vaginal or anal) or engage in any other sexual activity with a person who is under the age of 18 if a practitioner is in a 'position of trust' (as defined by the Act) in relation to that person. However, sexual abuse in the context of the nurse–patient relationship denotes broader range of acts than indicated by statute. The UKCC (1999) defines sexual abuse thus:

> Sexual abuse is forcing, inducing or attempting to induce the client to engage in any form of sexual activity. This encompasses both physical behaviour and remarks of a sexual nature that are made towards the client. Examples include touching the client inappropriately or engaging in sexual discussions which have no relevance to the client's care. (UKCC, 1999, p. 6)

Although some practitioners who sexually abuse patients may correspond to the popular image of the cold, calculating, self-gratifying sexual abuser, Green (1999) notes that there are a number of reasons why sexual abuse occurs, including:

- The perception of the practitioner that he or she is in love with the patient and that this takes precedence over other considerations.
- The practitioner may have a 'rescue fantasy' that is a belief that the patient can be rescued from suffering through a sexual relationship.
- The sexual contact occurs as both a manifestation of and contributing factor to serious mental breakdown on the part of the practitioner.

Improper actions may also be the consequence of misconceptions held by practitioners. Briant (1997) observes that some practitioners believe that it is acceptable to enter into a sexual relationship with a patient if the patient initiates the contact. This is, of course, incorrect. As already mentioned, the nurse–patient relationship is an example of a fiduciary relationship in which the parties concerned do not deal with each other on equal terms. The practitioner, as fiduciary, is generally in a more powerful position than the patient, and as such retains responsibility for controlling the boundaries of the relationship (Plaut, 1997; UKCC, 1999). Given the imbalance of power within fiduciary relationships, patients cannot be considered capable of consenting in a fully informed way to any personal relationship proposed by the fiduciary, nor can they be held responsible for a sexual relationship that they either initiate or permit to continue (Plaut, 1997). A further common misconception that Briant (1997) highlights is the belief that sexual relationships are permissible providing contact occurs outside the therapeutic environment or once direct clinical contact has ended. The UKCC (1999) states that personal relationships with vulnerable patients are never acceptable. Although it is acknowledged that illness and disability at any age can make people vulnerable, the UKCC (1999) acknowledges that some groups of patients and clients are more vulnerable to abuse than others. These include people who are physically frail, people with learning difficulties, people with mental health problems, and children. With regard to patients in general, it notes that the emotions aroused during a therapeutic relationship on part of either the patient or the practitioner, do not necessarily disappear as soon as the patient is discharged from care. Consequently, practitioners 'must carefully consider whether it is ever appropriate to have anything other than a purely professional relationship with a client or a former client' (UKCC, 1999, p. 8).

Preventing violations of the personal–professional boundary

According to Plaut (1997), probably the most important factor in preventing any violation of the personal–professional boundary is the practitioner's ability to be honest with him- or herself about whose needs are being met by the relationship. Although 'the only appropriate relationship between a client and practitioner is one that focuses exclusively upon the needs of the client' (UKCC, 1999, p. 4), Plaut (1997) acknowledges that many people enter caring or service professions because they need to be needed. This in itself is not problematic unless such needs are detrimental to patients, for example by delaying their recovery or preventing them from regaining full independence. The UKCC (1999) suggests that all practitioners should develop an understanding of the issues and processes whereby patients transfer expectations and experiences from the past on to practitioners and vice versa. The UKCC (1996b) recommends that all practitioners should have access to appropriate support and clinical supervision, which it defines as 'a practice-focussed professional relationship involving a practitioner reflecting on practice guided by a skilled supervisor'. It also advises that, with regard to the above, practitioners who work in isolation must be given particular consideration.

Plaut (1997) suggests that aspects of clinical relationships which may serve as risk factor or warning signs with regard to a possible breach of the personal–professional boundary include:

- Dual relationships conducted deliberately in private.
- Differential care or treatment provided for a patient without appropriate clinical justification.
- Loneliness or relationship difficulties in the practitioner's personal life.
- Constantly fantasizing about or looking forward to seeing a particular patient.
- Reluctance to discuss concerns about the relationship with colleagues or supervisors.

People are vulnerable whenever their health or usual function is impaired, but as the UKCC (1999) observes, some groups or patients are more vulnerable to abuse than others. In particular, patients who have a history of victimization or have suffered significant losses in their personal lives may be more at risk of becoming involved in a dual relationship that is detrimental to their well-being (Plaut, 1997).

Practitioners should remain alert to the possibility of patients misinterpreting comments or touch that are appropriate acts of care. Even simple clinical procedures may be misinterpreted and should therefore be explained to the patient before being carried out. Patients should be offered the opportunity to have a chaperone present during any intimate examination or procedure. Plaut (1997) suggests that if something questionable does happen, such as a possible misunderstanding or doubt about whether a particular act was appropriate or not, it is best not to keep knowledge of the event to oneself. He advocates documenting the incident in detail, seeking the opinion of a colleague or supervisor and, where appropriate, discussing any possible misunderstanding with the patient concerned.

Responding to sexual advances and sexual harassment

The potential for some aspects of nursing care to be perceived as sensual or sexually arousing is in part determined by how ill or well a patient is (Savage, 1987; Lawler, 1991). There is, for some patients, a point at which they are too unwell for nursing care to be construed as either a sensual or sexually arousing experience. Although there appears to be general acceptance among nurses that aspects of care may be sensual experiences for patients and possibly sexually arousing, situations where patients define nursing care as being primarily sexual are generally not tolerated by practitioners (Lawler, 1991). Thus, for example, a patient who deliberately exposes his erect penis will elicit a different response from a practitioner than the patient who has an involuntary erection during some aspect of intimate care.

On occasions patients may be attracted to those who nurse them and may express this attraction in the form of some sexual overture. Such advances may be consequence of:

- The patient's loneliness or lack of opportunity for any alternative form of sexual expression.
- The patient's need to seek confirmation of his or her attractiveness as a sexual being, which may have been undermined by illness or debility.
- The patient's need to 'deprofessionalize' the relationship, thereby rendering the practitioner powerless. This may indicate that the relationship is threatening aspects of the patient's self-concept or touches issues that are difficult for the patient.

Plaut (1997) suggests that a supportive exploration of what needs the patient is trying indirectly to express might be more beneficial to both the patient and the professional relationship than avoidance and distancing, confrontation or a simple recitation of the rules governing professional conduct. However, as Savage (1987) observes, there is a thin line between seductive behaviour and sexual harassment.

Defining exactly what constitutes sexual harassment is not easy. Robbins et al. (1997) observe that acts of sexual harassment are often ambiguous in nature, with innuendo and inappropriate touching predominating. Behaviour which is socially ambiguous is possibly more difficult for practitioners to respond to than overt sexual behaviour, such as deliberate exposure of the genitalia, the latter being easier to censure.

Patients who harass practitioners sexually are exploiting both the 'qualities' commonly associated with being a 'good nurse', such as kindness, friendliness, placing the needs of patients above one's own, and the conduct that is required of practitioners by their professional code. There is a general perception that a nurse is 'unable to leave the field because of her obligation to care for the patient' (Robbins et al., 1997) and some patients may try to exploit this. Practitioners may employ a number of strategies in response to patients' inappropriate behaviour, the chief among these being avoidance and distancing oneself from the perpetrator (Lawler, 1991; Finnis and Robbins, 1994; Guthrie, 1999). Robbins and colleagues (1997) suggest that sexual harassment is an abuse of power which, if it is to succeed, requires one or both of the two following conditions:

• A conspiracy of silence with the victim.
• Organizational collusion to inaction.

Consequently, any effective response to sexual harassment requires, at an individual level, support from colleagues and the opportunity for practitioners to communicate their experiences and subsequent feelings, and at an organizational level, a specific operational policy which includes a recognition of the legal right of an individual to pursue action through criminal prosecution where there has been a sexual assault (Robbins et al., 1997). The UKCC (1996a) states that no one should have to endure sexual harassment, and acknowledges in paragraph 17 of its *Guidelines for Professional Practice* that sexual harassment may constitute one of those situations where practitioners seek support or consider withdrawing care. It advises that 'any decision to withdraw care has to be taken very carefully and you should first discuss, if possible, the matter with managers, the patient's or client's family and, if appropriate and whenever possible, the patient or client themselves' (UKCC, 1996a, p. 12).

Key points of Chapter 2

• The nurse–patient relationship is a privileged relationship in which the practitioner accepts the confidence and trust of the patient to act at all times in the latter's best interests for the duration of that relationship.
• Establishing and maintaining appropriate professional boundaries is a necessity for effective psychosexual care. Boundaries enable both a

patient and a practitioner to engage safely in a therapeutic caring relationship.

- Professional behaviours which serve to create and maintain a therapeutic space in the nurse–patient relationship include maintaining confidentiality, recognizing and respecting the uniqueness and dignity of the patient, and avoiding violations of the personal–professional boundary.
- To promise a patient absolute confidentiality within the nurse–patient relationship is unethical as in certain very exceptional circumstances information may have to be disclosed with or without the patient's expressed consent.
- The recognition of a patient's sexuality is an essential aspect of respecting the uniqueness and dignity of the patient.
- Stereotyping patients inhibits psychosexual care.
- The only appropriate relationship with a patient is one that focuses exclusively on his or her health care needs. Personal relationships with patients inhibit psychosexual work and should not therefore be allowed to develop.
- Where practitioners and patients engage in a close therapeutic relationship, the potential for the relationship to develop in an improper manner increases.
- Practitioners undertaking psychosexual care should be alert to indicators of potential boundary violations in their professional relationships with patients and should have regular clinical supervision.
- No sexual contact should ever occur with a patient.

Key reading

Plaut, S.M. (1997) Boundary violations in professional–client relationships: overview and guidelines for prevention. *Sexual and Marital Therapy* **12**, 1, 77–94.
UKCC (1999) *Practitioner–client Relationships and the Prevention of Abuse*. London: United Kingdom Central Council for Nursing, Midwifery and Health Visiting.

CHAPTER 3

Psychosexual nursing skills

Introduction

Psychosexual nursing skills develop as the consequence of reflecting on the experiences and interactions practitioners have with patients, with each encounter between practitioner and patient being unique. Consequently, there can be no rigid formula or prescription as to how to respond to patients who are anxious or in distress. The psychosexual nursing skills required to provide psychosexual care are observation, listening, feeling, thinking and working collaboratively with patients to develop insight. Two aspects of the process of psychosexual care may be particularly helpful. The first of these relates to observation and listening and involves thinking about the extent to which the patient's general behaviour parallels his or her genital behaviour (Botell, 2001). The second is the capacity to think about the feelings that arise in the nurse–patient relationship in terms of the information they might provide as to how the patient is feeling and how he or she is experienced by others, particularly partners.

Observation

> The patient's appearance and behaviour provide clues which can be noted by the nurse, and used in an interpretative way with the patient. (Selby, 1989, p. 138)

Nurses, more than any other health professionals, have the most extended contact with patients within the health service. Consequently, they have greater opportunities to observe patients throughout their experiences of treatment and care. For this reason, it may well be to a nurse that a patient chooses to reveal his or her psychosexual anxiety or difficulties. Selby (1989) observes that as nurses are often the first person a patient meets in a

34

health care setting, they may become the recipient of inner tensions that the patient needs to express quickly. Conversely, nurses are often the last person in contact with a patient in many institutional settings and may end up 'picking up the pieces'. Between arrival and discharge, nurses are the professionals most likely to see patients at their private moments, in pain, exhausted, anxious or afraid (Green, 1999). Selby (1989) also suggests that nurses may be perceived by patients as less threatening and awe-inspiring than doctors. Patients may feel there is less 'distance' between nurses and themselves, and that practitioners are therefore more likely to understand the painful or possibly exciting feelings that they are experiencing.

Presenting behaviours

As discussed in Chapter 1, for a variety of reasons, many patients feel reluctant to mention directly their psychosexual problems and consequently the presentation of psychosexual distress is often indirect or covert. The recognition of psychosexual difficulties is therefore dependent to a large extent on the practitioner's ability to pick up on the 'cues' offered by the patient. Such 'cues' may take the form of the patient's 'presenting problem' or behaviours, the patient's non-verbal communication and the patient's response to intimate acts of care.

Examples of the possible indirect presentation of psychosexual problems include:

- Ruminating thoughts about sexually transmitted infections.
- Frequent visits to discuss methods of contraception.
- Unexplained genital symptoms.
- Complaints about partners.
- Persistent visits with seemingly minor or non-specific complaints.
- Reports of pain, depression or insomnia.

Although emotional pain may be converted into physical symptoms it is important that where a persistent physical symptom is described, any underlying pathology is excluded through appropriate medical examination and investigation. It is also important to guard against assuming that the behaviours listed above are always indicative of some 'deeper' psychosexual anxiety or distress and allowing this assumption to direct subsequent interactions with patients. Finally, any suggestion to the patient that his or her somatic symptoms may be indicative of emotional difficulties is likely to be rebuffed. According to Bor et al. (1998), possible reasons for this include:

- Some patients perceive physical symptoms to be more socially acceptable and less stigmatizing than psychological problems.
- Patients may prefer to view somatic symptoms as being entirely physical in origin as this seems to make problems more amenable to diagnosis and treatment.
- Somatic symptoms can have secondary gains for a patient in the form of attention he or she receives from both health professionals and non-professional care-givers.

Bor et al. (1998) suggest that pointing out these processes to the patient rarely alleviates the symptoms he or she is experiencing. It is possibly of greater benefit to the patient if a practitioner can create sufficient therapeutic space between herself and her patient (a process described later in this chapter), to enable the patient to discover his or her own unique connections between bodily symptoms and emotions (Penman, 1998). Other behaviours that may indicate the presence of psychosexual anxiety or distress include difficulties around attending appointments (*see* Chapter 1), the questions patients ask and the 'hints' patients make about their sexual relationships. Rogers (1989) is of the opinion that the patient who creates difficulties around getting or attending appointments may be indicating that he or she has something to communicate which they find difficult to acknowledge or embarrassing. Patients' behaviour with regard to attending appointments may also give some indication of what difficulties they may be experiencing in terms of maintaining an intimate relationship with others. Thus, increasing intimacy in the professional relationship with a practitioner may become too threatening for some patients, leading to their non-attendance or erratic attendance at subsequent appointments, until sufficient 'distance' has been restored. This 'dance of intimacy' may parallel that of the patient's relationship with his or her partner(s), or relationships with others in general.

Clifford (2000a) observes that when patients ask questions 'something tends to lie behind the question'. She notes that a tentative enquiry, such as *'Why do you ask?'*, is often worthwhile in addition to providing an answer. Patients may also drop hints of the psychosexual difficulties they may be experiencing in statements such as *'My partner and I are arguing all the time'* or *'She doesn't seem interested in me at the moment'*. Clifford (2000a) suggests that such statements are so vague that they could mean many things, but one possibility is that they may indicate some type of underlying sexual difficulty. Sometimes 'hints' may be even more indirect. Requests for screening for sexually transmitted infections, HIV testing or cervical cytology may all be 'presenting behaviours' for deeper psychosexual distress. Such requests draw the practitioner's attention to the patient's sexual behaviour and genitalia and may be an attempt to draw the practitioner's attention to some aspect of the patient's sexuality that feels disturbed or altered.

Non-verbal behaviour

Non-verbal communication commences immediately in any meeting between patient and practitioner. Selby (2001) notes that how a patient walks into a consultation, whether he or she is accompanied and how the patient responds to this person, as well as the things that a patient brings with him or her to a consultation, may all provide important clues to a patient's difficulties. Non-verbal communication is a particularly important source of information throughout the encounter. Examples of non-verbal behaviour, or body language, include:

- Posture and gesticulations.
- Facial expressions.
- General appearance in terms of grooming and dress.
- Observable autonomic physiological responses, such as blushing, pallor, quickened breathing and pupil dilation.

Egan (1990) observes that besides being a channel of communication in its own right, non-verbal behaviour often serves to punctuate or modify verbal communication. Non-verbal behaviours may:

- Confirm or repeat what is being communicated verbally.
- Contradict or obfuscate what is being communicated verbally.
- Strengthen or illuminate what is being communicated verbally.

Practitioners therefore need to remain aware not only of a patient's non-verbal behaviour during any consultation but also what *they may be communicating* non-verbally to their patient. According to Tomlinson (1998, p. 1573) aspects of patients' body language which may provide useful information during a consultation, include:

- Patients use of their hands and arms – behaviours such as twiddling with a ring or wringing of hands might indicate unease, as might defensively crossing arms or holding a bag or suitcase protectively on the lap.
- Pectoral flush, which creeps over the upper chest and neck, 'which indicates unease despite outward appearance of calm'.
- The way the patient positions him- or herself in the chair.
- 'Postural echo' or the mirroring of non-verbal behaviours between patient and practitioner. Tomlinson (1998) suggests that this occurs when there is 'harmony and empathy between the speakers'.

Where there is sometimes considerable discrepancy between what a patient is communicating verbally and non-verbally, it is often the non-verbal element of communication that is more accurate (Barton and Jewitt, 1995). Discomfort, as manifested by the non-verbal behaviour, may indicate that 'a person has something particularly important to discuss, such as an affair, anxiety about sexual anatomy, or acceptability of a particular form of sexual behaviour' (Hawton, 1985, p. 231). However, the patient's discomfort may also indicate that the practitioner has violated the patient's sense of privacy. It may be difficult for practitioners to know what the patient's non-verbal behaviour signifies. Reflecting back this sense of the patient's discomfort in a phrase such as *'I sense this might be uncomfortable for you'* acknowledges the patient's discomfort but leaves the control with the patient to indicate what is difficult about the situation and whether he or she wishes to explore this further.

Intimate care

> Doctors, midwives, nurses and physiotherapists have intimate physical contact with patients in their care. This means that they potentially disturb their patient's sense of their own private space even when they carry out the examination or treatment impeccably (Nicolson, 1998, p. 144)

The genital examination in psychosexual medicine is viewed as more than just a physical examination as it provides another avenue through which the patient's feelings and psychosexual anxieties can be explored (Skrine, 1989). However, as Selby (1989) notes, nurses, unlike doctors, generally do not examine patients genitally in order to make a diagnosis. There are occasions, however, where aspects of nursing care may provide practitioners with opportunities to observe for indicators of psychosexual distress. These may occur either during the provision of intimate nursing care, or when the practitioner is required to act as a chaperone. Intimate aspects of nursing care include:

- Inserting a urinary catheter.
- Bowel care.
- Dressing wounds in the genital area.
- Inserting suppositories and pessaries.
- Obtaining a cervical smear.
- Genital swabbing.
- Teaching the use of certain contraceptive devices such as diaphragms.
- Maintaining genital hygiene.

The vulnerability associated with such intimate aspects of care means that patients may reveal their distress or anxiety before, during or after such interventions. Practitioners need to be alert to how patients undress and position themselves on the couch, the patient's facial expression and what patients actually say – remarks such as *'I couldn't do what you do'* or *'I always hate this'* may have a significance beyond the context in which they occur. Whilst reactions may be expressed verbally, it is often the patient's non-verbal behaviour that is more revealing. Again, reflecting back what is sensed during such procedures though observations such as *'This appears difficult for you'*, provides the patient with an opportunity to explore such feelings further should he or she wish to do so. On occasions patients may find themselves suddenly and unexpectedly connected with past sexual experiences that have been traumatic. Such reawakened memories and the concomitant distress may be as great a shock to the patient as it is to the practitioner.

The recognition of anxiety or distress when revealed during such intimate procedures sometimes results in a patient being able to voice the 'fantasies' they have about their own genitalia. Wakley (1998) suggests that 'vaginal fantasies' occur frequently and include anxieties about the vagina being too small or too large, that its entrance is blocked or hidden, that the walls of the vagina are too rigid or fragile. The vagina may be viewed as something that is disgusting, dangerous or the conduit to a woman's insides or internal organs such as the liver, intestines and kidneys. Common 'penile fantasies' include that the penis is either too small or too large, that the penis can be 'broken' during sex. Wakley (1998) suggests such fantasies often emerge at the time of genital examination (or intimate care) and are not usually accessible by direct questioning. She cautions practitioners to:

Never jump to conclusions about people's fantasies on the basis of what you have
heard from others, or what you might have within yourself. Clever ideas prevent
patients explaining or exploring their own fantasies (Wakley, 1998, p. 151)

Practitioners who act as chaperones during genital examinations and
other intimate procedures also have opportunities to observe how the
patient may be feeling. Indeed, the chaperone may be better placed to
observe the patient's non-verbal behaviour as the person performing the
procedure may have 'distanced' him- or herself from the patient as a whole
in order to carry out the procedure (Meerabeau, 1999). The use of
chaperones is generally still contested, with some observers stating that
chaperones should always be present during intimate procedures for
medico-legal reasons (Bignell, 1999), whereas others feel that chaperones
should be offered rather than imposed on patients. Bignell (1999) writes
that most female patients want the offer of a chaperone and feel
uncomfortable asking for one if it is not offered, and that for women a
female nurse is generally the preferred choice. By contrast, male patients,
particularly young male patients, generally find the presence of a female
nurse as observer during their genital examination unwelcome. Beyond
the medico-legal implications, the function of chaperones is not well-
understood. Randall (1998) remarking on the work of doctors who practise
psychosexual medicine suggests that the presence of a third party
(chaperone) may impair psychosexual work by unbalancing the dynamics
of the consultation and making it less likely that a patient will articulate his
or her innermost fears or fantasies.

Offering to work with the patient

Clifford (1998b, p. 42) suggests that one of the tasks of practitioners is 'to
build bridges that patients may cross in safety to share their feelings'. The
first stage in this process is the recognition of psychosexual anxiety, pain
and distress; the next is conveying to the patient that his or her feelings are
a legitimate focus of consideration and care. This should always take the
form of a gentle invitation, which allows the patient to take his or her time,
delay any response, or refuse the offer. As Nichols (1993, p. 116) notes,
'You *offer* care, never force it. At the same time, note that you take the
initiative and do not wait for "something to come up" to precipitate your
action'.
     One way to make this invitation is to tentatively reflect back the sense of
distress that may be discernible from the patient's verbal and non-verbal
behaviour and ask whether there is anything else that is concerning the

patient, or which the patient wishes to discuss. The judicious and sensitive use of 'cue' questions, such as:

- *'How is love-making for you after the birth of your baby?'*
- *'How has your treatment affected your relationship with your partner?'*

conveys to patients that some people experience disturbances in their personal relationships at this point in time and that the practitioner is willing to listen and discuss any such difficulties as well as answer any questions the patient may have.

Communication skills

One of the key difficulties for both patient and practitioner associated with talking about sexual health is selecting the terms to be used to describe genitalia, sexual function and sexual activities. Hawton (1985, p. 103) advocates finding out what terms the patient understands and then trying to reach some common ground over the vocabulary to be used. He suggests that the use of correct medical and diagnostic terminology by patients should be viewed with caution as it may convey a shared understanding that does not truly exist. Patients may try to express their experiences in medical terms because they fear that the use of colloquialisms might cause offence, or they may fear appearing uninformed or ignorant. The use of vernacular terms by practitioners may also cause offence, may compromise professionalism and, like the use of medical terminology by patient and practitioner, may lead to an assumption about shared understanding that does not exist in reality. Bor and Watts (1993) conclude that it is best for practitioners to use simple, but not emotive terms, rather than obscure medical terminology, and to check out the patient's understanding of such terms, as even seemingly obvious expressions may not be understood.

Research suggests that a number of interactional strategies are often employed in clinical contexts to mark the use of 'delicate' items in conversations about sexual health. Such markers include disturbances in speech, such as pauses, hesitations and 'repairs' (when speakers correct their utterances), changes in intonation and body movements. Silverman and Perakyla (1990) refer to these interactional phenomena as 'perturbations'. It may be interesting for practitioners to note that Silverman and Perakyla (1990) observe that far from indicating difficulties in communication the use of perturbances are a necessary part of the interactional work required when talking about delicate issues.

The language a person uses often conveys the value system of the speaker. It is important to avoid terms that ascribe personal notions of normality or abnormality to aspects of the patient's sexuality (Bor and Watts, 1993). Similarly, it is important to avoid terms or phrases that convey presumptions about the patient. As Matthews (1998, p. 27) notes, 'Making inappropriate assumptions may render aspects of our patients' lives invisible to us, and this may well compromise our care'. In particular, practitioners need to ask 'neutral' questions that do not presume the gender of the patient's partner(s), the sexual orientation of the patient, or the nature or significance of the patient's relationships.

Generally, it is better to use 'open' questions, for example questions beginning with 'How', 'What' or 'When', rather than 'closed' questions as this gives the patient opportunities to express and expand upon any concerns. The judicious use of silence and repetition (repeating the last word or phrase the patient has used) may also enable the patient to expand upon what he or she is saying or to identify what is really bothering them. Paraphrasing or summarizing what the patient has said also serves a number of useful functions. It enables the practitioner to check out that he or she has actually heard the meaning of what the patient has said, it communicates this understanding to the patient and can help the patients to gather their thoughts when they appear to have become stuck (Egan, 1990; McNall, 2000).

The limitations of questions

Clifford (2000a, p. 50) observes that health professionals have become so used to collecting clinical information by means of questions and answers that this method of working with patients is in danger of prevailing in every encounter with patients. There are a number of difficulties with the use of questions in psychosexual care. The first is summarized by Wakley (1998) who writes:

> If you ask a lot of questions you get a lot of answers – but you may not hear what the problem is because you have not allowed the patient to tell you. (Wakley, 1998, p. 149)

The second difficulty is contained within Smith's (1989) observation that:

> The conventional approach, based on eliciting factors by questioning and then telling the patient what to do, is inadequate in a situation where feelings are the underlying cause of the patient's difficulty; for a patient in a state of confused feeling may well feel even more confused after undergoing prolonged questioning that yields understanding and medical instructions that promise no relief. (Smith, 1989, p. 37)

The observations made by Wakley (1998) and Smith (1989) indicate some of the potential limitations of the 'question and answer' format in the process of psychosexual care. A number of other issues also need to be considered with regard to the role of information-gathering in the process of psychosexual care. The first of these is described by John Bancroft in an interview with Dryden (1985) and relates to the ethics of collecting a large amount of very sensitive and personal information from people which may not be of any use to the patient's care. De Raeve (1998, p. 138) writes that practitioners need not only to respect patients' privacy but also to protect it actively from invasive inquiries and from the practitioner's own curiosity. Furthermore, the asking a series of formal questions may convey to the patient that the solution to the patient's difficulties lies outside of the patient and is in the gift of 'experts'. Reverting to asking a series of questions may indicate the practitioner's 'flight' from the uncomfortable or disturbing feelings that are in the 'here and now' of the nurse–patient relationship.

When thinking about the role of questioning in helping patients who are experiencing psychosexual distress, it is useful to remember Clifford's (2000a) contention that the aim of questioning is understanding, not the desire to know or the need to find out. Such understanding is often best achieved by listening rather than questioning, and remaining 'unknowing' when faced by a patient who is anxious, confused or distressed.

The value of 'unknowing'

Clifford (2000b, p. 2) states that practitioners' expectations that they should 'know' is often a handicap to the professional skills required when encountering a patient who is experiencing emotional or psychosexual difficulties. She suggests that such 'knowing' can potentially both prevent understanding what the patients might be actually seeking and deny patients space to think about and articulate their feelings and explore what they wish to do. Penman (1998) elaborates on how the dynamics of the nurse–patient relationship may militate against 'unknowing'. She notes that when practitioners are perceived as or act as 'experts', the patient is generally not invited to offer an understanding of his or her problems as there is an expectation that the 'expert', with access to theoretical and professional knowledge, will generate a solution. Practitioners may also refer to theoretical constructs, personal ideals and assumptions based on previous clinical and personal experiences to 'comfort' a patient and in doing so smother any expression of his or her distress. Consequently, neither practitioner nor patient has the opportunity to 'hear' the extent and nature of the patient's feelings. It is important, therefore, for practitioners to refrain from offering information, advice and reassurance, no matter how well-meaning, until the problem is fully understood by both patient and practitioner (Selby, 1989; Wakley, 1998). Fabricius (1991, p. 102) recalls an observation made by a 'wise and experienced principal tutor' who pointed out that 'reassuring the patient was like isolating a fire with a fire-blanket – it stopped you catching alight too and left the patient burning alone'.

However, remaining 'unknowing' is a difficult position for practitioners to hold as it may generate feelings of vulnerability and uselessness in the practitioner. As Selby (1989, p. 143) observes, 'tolerating this feeling of uselessness is one of the most important skills to be learned'. It is also one of the most difficult as it requires the practitioner to refrain from activities that help nurses to feel in charge of the situation and enjoying the satisfaction that providing patients with professional knowledge usually brings. Practitioners may defend themselves against the pain of not knowing what to do, by reassurance, giving advice or perhaps unthinkingly referring-on.

Conversely, according to Penman (1998), if practitioners allow themselves not to know, or presume to know, the answer to a patient's difficulties, the practitioner is able to observe the information the patient is able to offer. Penman (1998) suggests that the patient is 'freed' by this unknowing to become aware of his or her own pain and distress, and the protective barriers that cause psychosexual difficulties, that is, to discover the connections between feelings and their somatic or behavioural symptoms. The nurse–patient relationship becomes a process of collaborative enquiry which recognizes that patients have within themselves the information necessary to resolve their own difficulties and at the same time creates space for them to explore their own feelings.

Thinking about the nurse–patient relationship

Thinking about the interaction between nurse and patient may provide some insight into the patient's difficulties. During the process of collaborative enquiry, the practitioner is required not only to listen to what the patient is feeling and experiencing but also to think about what is happening in the 'here and now' (Selby, 1989). The key to thinking about the 'here and now' is developing an awareness of feelings. As Clifford (2000b, p. 4) remarks, 'recognizing feelings evoked in clinical work gives our patients and us the opportunity for more useful and rewarding work together'. Conversely, unrecognized feelings may actually interrupt or stop work with a patient. There are a number of difficulties associated with working with feelings. First, feelings do not usually constitute the focus of most practitioners' training. Second, there is what Clifford (2000a, p. 75) terms a learned 'hierarchy of morality in feelings' that represses and prevents the recognition of certain feelings that have come to be seen as unacceptable in relationships with patients. Such feelings may include anger, disgust and hate, and may be difficult for patients and practitioners alike to acknowledge and subsequently may become problematic for patients and practitioners to deal with.

Practitioners can sometimes use their own feelings to clarify what is happening for the patient. This use of the practitioner's feelings can represent a powerful way of gaining deeper understanding for patient and practitioner alike, when this does not arise in the verbal interaction of the nurse–patient relationship. In order to do this, practitioners need to be able to recognize and accept their feelings, no matter how unacceptable or unwelcome they might seem. Practitioners also need to think about whether these feelings could be a reflection of how the patient is feeling and to contemplate what it might feel like for the patient to be experiencing such feelings. Finally, this needs to be explored with the patient.

In order to work in this way with patients, practitioners need sufficient self-awareness to discern whether feelings that arise during clinical encounters are the consequence of resonances of their own personal experiences that are evoked by aspects of the patient or his or her circumstances. Sometimes what the practitioner feels during an encounter with a patient may be the complement to the patient's expressed feelings, that is, the practitioner witnesses the whole meaning of what the patient is communicating when the patient can only afford to acknowledge a part. In other words, the practitioner feels 'what is missing' from the patient's awareness. The practitioner may also feel what other people (including the patient's partner) experience when they encounter the patient, thereby gaining some information about the patient's possible interpersonal difficulties. On some occasions, patients may subconsciously project difficult or disturbing feelings on to practitioners and practitioners who are able to recognize a patient's pain and distress, may 'hold' some of that pain and distress for a patient (Fabricius, 1991). This may be therapeutic as it helps to make such feelings seem less overwhelming and therefore more manageable to the patient. Often, projected feelings seem to 'come out of nowhere' in that they are incongruous with what is going on at the general level of interaction with a patient. The intensity of the emotion felt during such a consultation may give a practitioner some idea as to the strength and possible unacceptability (to the patient) of the feelings that the patient is experiencing.

Recognition of difficult feelings can be shared sensitively and judiciously with a patient using reflection: *'I can hear a great deal of anger / sadness / pain, etc., in your voice at the moment'*; a tentative exploration: *'I sense there seems to be something that is difficult for you about this conversation'*; or a combination of these approaches: *'I feel confused at the moment, I wonder if this is how you may be feeling?'*. It is important to acknowledge distress and allow patients time to explore what they are feeling in such situations. Acknowledging difficult feelings evoked in clinical encounters gives both patients and nurses opportunities to develop insight into the patient's difficulties. In order to do this, practitioners are required sometimes to act as a 'container' for the patient's projections (Fabricius, 1991). This means abandoning the comfort of offering reassurance (offering reassurance is viewed by Fabricius (1991) as a refusal to accept the patient's projections) and being prepared 'not only to listen to and feel with the patient, but also to be able to think about what is happening in the "here and now" ' (Selby, 1989, pp 140–141).

Referral

Selby (2001) considers that in psychosexual nursing it is always worth trying 'to stay' with the patient rather than referring him or her and to try to become aware of the defences in both oneself and the patient which may hinder or halt therapeutic work. It is also important, however, that practitioners recognize their own limitations and those of their patients. Where the feelings and thoughts a patient describes seem to indicate underlying mental ill-health or long-standing personality problems, referral should be made to appropriate members of the mental health care team. Similarly, with patients presenting with persisting impairment of sexual function, practitioners will need to discuss the importance of seeking a medical opinion (as altered sexual response may sometimes be an indicator of underlying physical pathology) and the possibility of referral for psychosexual counselling or therapy (*see* Chapter 5). Where persisting relationship problems are identified, referral to Relate should be considered.

Balanced against the importance of recognizing one's own limitations, needs to be an awareness of the defensive function of referral. Selby (1989) suggests that if a nurse invariably refers when the patient indicates there is a problem, this may act as defence against becoming involved. Ideally, any referral should only occur when both patient and practitioner have had sufficient opportunity to gain an understanding of what the patient's difficulties actually are. On occasions, a problem shared may be all that is required.

Glover (1985) notes that occasionally if the relationship between patient and nurse has existed for a considerable period of time, a referral may be perceived as a threat (by both patient and practitioner) in that it may be interpreted as rejection or a sign of failure. Some patients may have previously had psychosexual, relationship or general counselling, sometimes over a considerable period of time, and it is important to establish why this was not satisfactory before making another referral (Selby, 2001). Practitioners need to be aware of what agencies are available locally, the nature and availability of services that are offered, the training and supervision of staff who work for the agency, and how patients can access such services.

Continuing training and support

Clifford (2000a) suggests that this type of emotional labour requires continuing training in working with feelings that arise from clinical encounters and on-going support for practitioners. Clifford (2000a, p. 119) states that 'the practitioner's experience of being recognized as an individual, understood and acknowledged, supports a standard of sensitive care that enhances the way in which patients, partners and relatives are cared for'. Possible opportunities for practitioners to study their own clinical work include structured seminar training groups, such as Balint-style psychosexual seminar groups (Clifford, 1998a; Penman, 1998; Selby, 2000), more informally structured 'specialist interest' groups and clinical supervision. Fabricius (1991, p. 103) suggests that the demands patients make on practitioners in terms of the feelings they project – both in terms of quantity and intensity – are too much for practitioners unless practitioners themselves are held in a supporting containing structure.

Key points of Chapter 3

- The process of psychosexual care entails the recognition of psychosexual anxiety and distress and creating opportunities for patients to share their feelings.
- In addition to helping to create a therapeutic space in which a patient may begin to develop an understanding of the links between his or her feelings and psychosexual difficulties, the practitioner also needs to think about the feelings that arise within the nurse–patient relationship and how awareness of such feelings may be used to help the patient.
- Observation of, and reflection on, the patient's appearance, presenting behaviours and non-verbal communication may help both the patient and practitioner to develop a better understanding of the patient's difficulties. Practitioners should consider the extent to which the patient's general behaviour parallels the patient's genital behaviour.
- Although emotional pain may be converted into physical symptoms it is important that patients with persisting physical symptoms attend for appropriate medical examination and investigation.
- Suggesting to patients directly that somatic symptoms are the consequence of emotional difficulties is likely to be rejected by the patient.
- Intimate aspects of care often provide useful insights to the patient's feelings as this is when patients are most likely to voice their 'fantasies' or anxieties about their genitalia or sexual activities.
- Reflecting back to the patient the sense of distress discernible in her or his verbal and non-verbal communication, and the sensitive use of 'cue' questions may convey to the patient that his or her feelings are legitimate focus for consideration and care.
- Information-gathering, sexual history taking and offering reassurance and advice are unlikely to help the patient where feelings are the cause of the patient's difficulties.
- The practitioner who remains 'unknowing' when faced by a patient in distress is one who desists from offering 'expert opinion' in the form of information based on professional theories or previous clinical experience, or 'comfort' in the form of reassurance, before the patient's problem has been fully understood.
- This 'unknowing', in turn, creates a space for the patient to become more aware of his or her feelings and to develop an understanding of the

relationship between these feelings and the difficulties he or she may be experiencing.

- Thinking about what is happening both in terms of behaviour and feelings arising in the 'here and now' of the nurse–patient relationship may generate information which when shared with patients can enable them to resolve their own psychosexual difficulties in a way that suits them best.

- A practitioner's ability to 'hold' the distress of the patient is in part determined by whether the practitioner works within a supportive and containing structure. Working with feelings that arise within and as a consequence of clinical work requires practitioners to have access to continuing training and ongoing support.

Key reading

Clifford, D. (2000a) Section 1 Developing psychosexual awareness. In: Wells, D. (ed.). (2000) *Caring for Sexuality in Health and Illness*. Edinburgh: Churchill Livingstone; chapters 1–6.

Selby, J. (1989) Psychosexual nursing. In: Skrine, R.L. (ed.). Introduction to Psychosexual Medicine. Carlisle: Montana Press.

CHAPTER 4

Altered sexual interest and response

Introduction

Some patients that practitioners encounter will complain of altered sexual interest and/or response. Although each individual patient is unique in terms of the significance and meaning that he or she will attribute to such changes, it is important that practitioners have some awareness of the many physical, psychological and interpersonal factors that may alter sexual response. Undoubtedly, the majority of people practitioners will encounter in their day-to-day clinical practice will be experiencing alterations in sexual interest and response that are related to changes in health, and the focus of this chapter in part reflects this bias. Ill-health and disability may result in changes to sexual interest and response in a variety of ways (*see* Bancroft, 1989, pp 552–553). These include:

- The physical effects of the condition – both specific interference with genital or other sexual responses (particularly so with endocrine, neurological and cardiovascular conditions) and non-specific effects, such as pain, fatigue and immobility.
- The effects of treatment on sexual interest and response, including the side-effects of certain drugs, the damage caused by surgery or trauma either directly to the genitalia or to the neurological and vascular control of genital response, and the psychological effects of altered body image.
- The psychological effects of the condition, or treatments used, on the individual and the individual's partner(s).

Often many changes in sexual response, be they health-related or not, will be only temporary (although no less distressing for many who experience them); however, sometimes such changes persist, becoming sexual dysfunctions (*see* Chapter 5).

Sexual response

Sexual function has been described as a process that is essentially 'psychosomatic', that is, the consequence of an interplay between psychological and somatic events (Bancroft, 1989). Murphy (1998) provides a useful review of the complex biology of human sexual response. He notes that whilst there has been considerable investigation of the neuro-endocrine mechanisms of sexual desire and arousal in male mammals and of the biological mechanisms of human penile erection, there has been much less research investigating the biological basis of sexual desire and response in females. Consequently, it is questionable as to how far what is known about the biology of sexual desire and arousal can be generalized to women.

The female and male physiological changes that occur during sexual arousal are dependent on two processes: vasocongestion and myotonia. Vasocongestion in the genital area causes the genitals to swell and change colour. This increased concentration of blood in the genital areas is also accompanied by increased muscle tension (myotonia). If orgasm is attained, involuntary muscle contraction occurs followed by relaxation. Various models have been proposed to describe the human pattern of sexual response, the best-known being that delineated by Masters and Johnson (1966) in the book *Human Sexual Response*.

Masters and Johnson (1966) divide the physical and physiological changes that occur in sexual response into four stages:

- Excitement.
- Plateau.
- Orgasm.
- Resolution.

Some commentators have subsequently suggested that an additional stage – sexual desire – precedes this pattern of sexual response (Kaplan, 1977).

Sexual desire

Sexual desire may be triggered by both external cues (sight, smell, sound and taste) and internal cues (thoughts, fantasies, certain emotions). It is influenced by hormonal, neurological and physiological factors and also by what Daines and Perrett (2000, p. 15) describe as 'an emotional and psychological energy that is relationship seeking'. Daines and Perrett (2000) suggest that this aspect of desire is shaped profoundly by intrapsychic issues and relationships with others, including the society in which an individual lives. Spence (1991, p. 13) conceptualizes sexual desire in a more behaviourist paradigm as 'a drive state in which a need is created to engage in a particular behaviour, in this case sexual behaviour, in order to reduce the "need" or drive state'. Spence (1991) observes that desire cannot be equated simply with the frequency of sexual arousal or activity, given that desire may occur in the absence of sexual arousal and activity. She also notes that although a distinction tends to be made between sexual arousal and sexual desire, the relationship between these two aspects of the human sexual response is not as clear-cut as some commentators have suggested (see also Basson, 2001).

Excitement

This is a response to sexual stimulation – either through fantasy or in reality – which marks the start of the physical and physiological changes associated with sexual arousal. Sexual arousal is usually accompanied by a number of somatic changes in both sexes, including raised heart rate, elevated blood pressure, increased muscular tension and changes to the skin. The vagina usually becomes very moist with lubricant produced by the vaginal mucosal lining. The inner two-thirds of the vagina expands and distends as the vaginal walls swell and open up. The labia majora may separate and increase in diameter and the labia minora may thicken and expand as the consequence of vasocongestion. The increase in blood flow also affects the uterus, which both expands and tilts both up and forward from the pelvic floor. The head of the clitoris may swell and the shaft of the clitoris may elongate. The nipples of some women's breasts may also become erect.

Hawton (1985, p. 13) notes that although the physical changes during sexual excitement may proceed steadily, some womens' subjective experience of the sexual excitement phase is that of 'a series of waves of increasing and decreasing sexual arousal or tension'. For many women the intensity of feelings experienced during the excitement phase will also vary greatly between one sexual experience and another.

In men, erection of the penis occurs as the consequence of penile arterial dilation, increased arterial blood supply, active relaxation of the smooth muscle tissue of the corpora cavernosa and constriction of venous outflow, thereby enabling the penis to become engorged and erect. The scrotal sac tightens, elevating the testes and in uncircumcised men the foreskin usually retracts; nipple erection may also occur in some men. The increase in the size of the penis during erection is not directly proportional to the size of the penis when it is flaccid and the size and firmness of erections often fluctuate considerably during sexual arousal (Hawton, 1985).

Plateau phase

This describes the excitement phase as it continues to the brink of orgasm for women and the point of ejaculatory inevitability for men. For some women vaginal distension will continue during this phase with the outer third of the vagina swelling and therefore narrowing the entrance to the vagina. The clitoral shaft and glans retract to the extent that the clitoris withdraws fully under the clitoral hood and lies up against the pubic symphysis. Breast enlargement and areolar engorgement may also occur at this stage. During the plateau phase in the male sexual response, the penis undergoes further enlargement which is confined mostly to the coronal ridge of the glans penis which may also change colour.

Orgasm

It is thought that orgasm in women is triggered by a neural reflex arc in response to pronounced genital vasocongestion. Women who have experienced orgasm describe a sensation that comes in waves of feeling as the uterus, vaginal and pelvic floor muscles contract rhythmically. Not all women are aware of these contractions. Often, this sensation is preceded by a sense of 'orgasmic inevitability'. In women who do experience orgasm, the concomitant sensations and feelings may vary in intensity from one occasion to another. As the sexual response of women does not include a refractory period, some women may experience one orgasm quickly followed by another (or others) without loss of arousal.

The orgasm phase in men is preceded by a distinct sense of 'ejaculatory inevitability', that is, the point at which it feels that ejaculation cannot be averted. The sensation of ejaculatory inevitability is thought to be the result of contractions of the accessory sex organs – the prostate gland and seminal vesicles – which in turn lead to an emission of seminal fluid into the prostatic urethra. Emission of the ejaculate is the consequence of contractions in the epididymus, vas deferens, seminal vesicles and prostate during which the internal sphincter of the bladder is closed, thereby preventing retrograde ejaculation. For most men the subjective experience of orgasm occurs at the emission stage and is most intense during ejaculation.

Resolution

During this phase the anatomical and physiological changes associated with earlier phases of sexual response are reversed and the body returns to its unaroused state. In the male sexual response the resolution phase also includes a 'refractory period', that is, a time during which further ejaculation is not possible. The duration of this period may vary from minutes to hours, but tends to increase with age.

Limitations of the human sexual response cycle

This conceptualization of the different phases of sexual response in men and women is based on clinical observations made by Masters and Johnson (1966) of the physiological responses of sexually aroused subjects in a laboratory setting and has its limitations. Tiefer (1991) highlights some important methodological weaknesses associated with the original research that underpins 'the human sexual response cycle' (HSRC) model. Tiefer (1991, p. 5) concludes that the original research of Masters and Johnson (1966) 'was designed to identify physiological functions of subjects experienced with particular preselected sexual responses' and that 'rather than the HSRC being the best-fit model chosen to accommodate their research, the HSRC actually guided the selection of subjects for the research'. This not only compromises the generalizability of this model of human sexual response, but 'imposes a false biological uniformity on sexuality which does not support the human uses and meanings of sexual potential' (Tiefer, 1991, p. 20). Savage (1987, p. 13) points out that the emphasis placed on attaining an orgasm within the Masters and Johnson (1966) model means that sexual response is 'framed as goal-orientated, to the extent that sexual fulfilment has become entirely synonymous with orgasm'. Savage (1987) further notes that although the pattern of the Masters and Johnson (1966) model is a simplification, it has become a template for many people's expectations of what they should experience. Savage (1987, p. 14) concludes that the Masters and Johnson (1966) model is 'based on a drive theory of sexuality in which the biological nature of sexual motivation is seen to be as compelling as the need for food and drink. It fails to do justice to the *meaning* that sexual acts hold for individuals or for their emotional associations'. Thus, Savage (1987) issues the following caution with regard to the sharing of information derived from the research of Masters and Johnson (1966) with patients:

> Masters and Johnson have given us a wealth of information about the physiology of sexual response. And there is no doubt that poor theoretical knowledge of anatomy and physiology can, in part, be the cause of an unsatisfying sexual relationship. But reading a text book will not necessarily inform anyone of the particular needs of a specific partner. (Savage, 1987, p. 14)

Ill-health, disability and sexual response

It is known that a number of disease processes, surgical interventions and drugs are associated with alterations in sexual interest and response. Some of the medical conditions that may lead to changes in sexual interest and function include the following:

Adrenal disease

Adrenal insufficiency (Addison's disease) is associated with impaired sexual interest (a probable consequence of reduced androgen production) and less frequent orgasm in women affected by this condition. Impaired sexual interest has also been noted in men with adrenal insufficiency. Adrenal overactivity (Cushing's syndrome) sometimes increases and sometimes diminishes women's sexual interest, although often it remains unaffected. Many men, however, experience impaired sexual interest and erectile problems (Hawton, 1985).

Cardiovascular disease

Up to 25% of men with erectile problems may have some form of vascular lesion that is compromising erectile function. Murphy (1998) states that evidence of peripheral vascular disease, hypertension, a history of CVA or ischaemic heart disease, diabetes mellitus, obesity and smoking should alert clinicians to this possibility. Vascular occlusion of the bifurcation of the aorta may cause erectile problems that are the consequence of claudication. Arteriosclerotic changes and thrombus formation in the internal iliac, internal pudendal and penile arteries are often associated with the insidious onset of a gradual decline in the ability to attain and maintain an erection. Bancroft (1989) notes that several studies have shown that there is a persisting decline in sexual activity after myocardial infarction (*see also* Jones and Nugent, 2001; Kelly, 2001) but also reports that there are some data that suggest sexual dysfunction is unusually prevalent in both men and women preceding a heart attack. Studies of women and men following coronary bypass surgery suggest that in women it is sexual interest that is most likely to be affected, whereas in men it is sexual arousal (Bancroft, 1989).

Chronic renal failure

Bancroft (1989) reports that women and men with chronic renal failure have a high prevalence of sexual problems. He notes that in some studies 90% of men and 80% of women have reported reduced sexual interest and that similar proportion complained of erectile problems or, in women, of impaired arousal and difficulties reaching orgasm.

Diabetes

Murphy (1998) notes that erectile problems have been reported in 34–75% of diabetic men, but only a minority of men have erectile problems at the initial clinical presentation of hyperglycaemia and, in many of these men, erectile function improves with insulin treatment. The two organic factors of most importance in diabetes-related erectile dysfunction are arterial insufficiency and peripheral neuropathy (Murphy, 1998). Murphy (1998) remarks that there is no entirely reliable way of establishing which erectile problems are caused by arterial insufficiency rather than psychological factors, although he claims that the loss of nocturnal penile tumescence strongly suggests the former. The persistence of nocturnal penile tumescence, however, should not entirely rule out the possibility of a vascular cause. Less is known about the effects of diabetes on the sexual response of women, although a few studies have suggested that diabetic women may experience more difficulties with arousal and orgasm (Berman and Berman, 2001).

Epilepsy

A number of studies have drawn attention to the high frequency of lowered sexual interest, less frequent sexual intercourse and arousal difficulties in people with temporal lobe epilepsy, although overall there is a wide variation in the reported rates of sexual dysfunction in people with epilepsy.

Genitourinary conditions

Genitourinary conditions, such as imperforate hymen, vulvodynia, Peyronie's disease, prostatitis, priapism and sexual infections (*see* Chapter 8) may all contribute to difficulties in sexual function.

Hypogonadism

This is often the result of conditions, such as mumps orchitis, undescended testes, pituitary tumours, cirrhosis and Klinefelter's syndrome. In women it also occurs as the result of natural menopause. If hypogonadism is severe in men, it may result in loss of sexual interest, erectile dysfunction and ejaculatory failure (Hawton, 1985). Butcher (1999) notes that loss of sexual interest in some women may occur as a result of 'androgen deficiency syndrome' secondary to hysterectomy with bilateral salpingo-oophorectomy or cytotoxic chemotherapy.

Hypopituitarism

Sexual dysfunction associated with hypopituitarism results from hypogonadotrophic hypogonadism (Hawton, 1985). Impaired sexual interest and orgasmic dysfunction are common problems in women affected by this condition, and men often experience impaired sexual interest, erectile and ejaculatory problems.

Hyperprolactinaemia

Hyperprolactinaemia impairs gonadal function and has been associated with impairment of sexual interest, erectile dysfunction and a decrease in the orgasmic frequency in women.

Hypothalamo-pituitary disease

Murphy (1998) reports that numerous clinical case reports identify loss of sexual interest and failure of arousal with structural lesions of the hypothalamus. He notes that these include sexual problems which are not explained by endocrine function nor ameliorated by hormone replacement.

Multiple sclerosis

The most commonly reported alterations in sexual response reported by women are decreased sensation, decreased sexual interest, decreased frequency or loss of orgasm and difficulties with arousal. Erectile problems are the most frequently reported problem of men with multiple sclerosis, followed by decreased sensation, decreased sexual interest and ejaculatory problems.

Peripheral nerve lesions

Damage to the pelvic plexus during surgery such as radical cystectomy, abdomino-perineal resection of the rectum and radical retro-pubic prostatectomy, can cause erectile problems. Damage may also occur during trans-urethral prostatectomy, drainage of prostatic abscesses, external sphincterotomy and internal urethrotomy (Murphy, 1998). Less is known at present about the effects of hysterectomy and other gynaecological surgery on the pelvic plexus in women, although some commentators observe that injury to the utero-vaginal and cervical plexus during hysterectomy may have an adverse effect on sexual arousal and orgasm (Berman and Berman, 2001).

Spinal cord injury

Reflex erections continue to occur in some men with complete transection of the spinal cord above the sacral segments despite an absence of penile sensation. If the sacral cord is damaged, reflex erections are lost, but some people claim that psychogenic erections (that is, erections in response to sexual thoughts) can still occur (Murphy, 1998). In some men with spinal cord injuries above T6, sexual stimulation may lead to excessive excitation of the autonomic nervous system as signals travelling up the spinal column become blocked at the level of the lesion. This leads to the activation of local vasoconstriction responses which cause a rapid rise in blood pressure, leading to intense headache. Responses from the parasympathetic nervous system to lower blood pressure cannot travel down the spinal cord beyond the lesion so blood pressure continues to rise. This phenomena is sometimes referred to as 'autonomic dysreflexia' and if untreated may result in convulsions, cerebral haemorrhage and death (Glass and Soni, 1999). Few data are available that detail the effects of spinal cord injuries on the female sexual response, although what material does exists, suggests that sexual response in women with spinal injuries is somewhat less affected than it is in men (Bancroft, 1989).

Thyroid disease

Erectile dysfunction is a common occurrence in men with hyperthyroidism (thyrotoxicosis) and occasionally hypersexuality occurs in

Table 4.1: Possible sexual side-effects of some commonly prescribed medications

Altered sexual interest:
    Anti-convulsants: phenytoin, primidone
    Anti-depressants: (tricyclic) amitriptyline, amoxapine, clomipramine, imipramine,
    maprotiline, nortriptyline, (monoamine oxidase inhibitors), phenelzine
    Anti-psychotics: chlorpromazine, fluphenazine
    Anti-hypertensives: labetalol, methyldopa, metoprolol, propranolol, timolol
    Anti-emetics: metoclopramide
    Anti-cholinergics: diphenhydramine, hydroxyzine
    Benzodiazepines
    Hormonal methods of contraception
    Barbiturates
Erectile dysfunction:
    Anti-convulsants: carbamazepine, phenytoin, primidone
    Anti-depressants: (tricyclics) amitriptyline, amoxapine, clomipramine, imipramine,
    maprotiline, nortriptyline; (monoamine oxidase inhibitors) phenelzine, (selective serotonin
    re-uptake inhibitors) fluoxetine, fluvoxamine, paroxetine, sertraline
    Anti-psychotics: chlorpromazine, fluphenazine, haloperidol, thioridazine
    Anti-hypertensives: atenolol, clonidine, hydralazine, methyldopa, metoprolol, pindolol,
    propanolol, timolol, verapamil
    Anti-emetics: metoclopramide
    Anti-cholinergics: diphenhydramine, hydroxyzine, propantheline, scopolamine
    Anti-spasmodics: baclofen
    Benzodiazepines
    Diuretics: amiloride, chlortalidone, indapamide, spironolactone, bendroflumethiazide
    Hypolipidaemics: bezafibrate, gemfibrozil, fenofibrate
    Barbiturates
    Non-steroidal anti-inflammatory: naproxen
Delayed/absence of ejaculation:
    Anti-depressants: amitriptyline, amoxapine, clomipramine, imipramine, phenelzine,
    fluoxetine, fluvoxamine, paroxetine, sertraline
    Anti-hypertensives: clonidine, guanethidine, labetalol, methyldopa, propranolol
    Anti-psychotics: chlorpromazine, fluphenazine, haloperidol, thioridazine
    Anti-spasmodics: baclofen
    Benzodiazepines
    Barbiturates
    Non-steroidal anti-inflammatory: naproxen
Delayed/absence of orgasm:
    Anti-depressants: clomipramine, imipramine, phenelzine
    Anti-hypertensives: clonidine, methyldopa, propranolol
    Anti-psychotics: thioridazine
    Benzodiazepines

Based on information from Murphy (1998) and Tomlinson (1998)

both men and women affected by this condition. Impaired sexual interest is seen in the majority of men and women affected by hypothyroidism. Some women with hypothyroidism also experience difficulties with orgasm and erectile dysfunction may occur in some men (Hawton, 1985).

Surgical interventions may adversely affect sexual response either directly through trauma done to the peripheral nervous system (particularly associated with bowel, genital and pelvic surgery) or through the alteration caused to an individual's body image. Conversely, surgical intervention may improve sexual expression in some individuals if painful or debilitating symptoms are alleviated, or fear of life-threatening conditions is reduced or eliminated by such interventions. Unsurprisingly, treatment for gynaecological cancers, breast, testicular and prostatic cancers and surgery resulting in the formation of a stoma is associated with a high incidence of psychosexual sequelae (Cull et al., 1993; Crowther, et al. 1994; Champion, 1996; Huish et al., 1998; Hartmann et al., 1999). Certain forms of surgery remove all possibility of undertaking certain sexual acts. Abdomino-perineal resection of the rectum may not only lead to erectile and ejaculatory problems in some men, and loss of sensation, lack of vaginal secretions and dyspareunia for some women, but also removes a source of sexual satisfaction for men and women who enjoy receptive anal intercourse.

Although the information given above is not exhaustive, it should be sufficient to alert practitioners to the importance of referring patients who present with a persisting impairment of sexual response for appropriate medical examination and clinical investigation (*see* Friedman, 1988; Dean, 1998). Although the findings of medical examination are often entirely normal, Dean (1998) argues that the reassurance offered by this can be an important factor in an individual's recovery of his or her 'sexual well-being'. Practitioners need also to be aware that the lack of training in sexual medicine for doctors at undergraduate level may mean, however, that some of their medical colleagues are ill-prepared for the management of patients with sexual difficulties (Adler, 1998). Practitioners also need to be aware of the work of clinical nurse specialists and their importance in helping to prevent adverse psychosexual sequelae in patients undergoing gynaecological, breast, urological and stoma surgery, through pre- and post-operative education, counselling and support (*see* Huish et al., 1998; Maughan and Clarke, 2001).

Medical and recreational drugs

The possible side-effects of some prescribed medications are known to include changes in sexual functioning (*see* Table 4.1).

The list of medications in Table 4.1 is not exhaustive and practitioners should always refer to the *British National Formulary* and the pharmaceutical manufacturer's datasheets with regard to the possible effects of any particular medication on sexual functioning. It is impossible to predict accurately how any one individual will respond to a particular drug, including what, if any, effect it may have on his or her sexual response. When trying to appraise the likelihood of 'a drug-induced sexual effect', Bancroft (1989, pp 600–601) suggests that clinicians need to ask the following questions:

- What proportion of people taking the drug are affected this way?
- How specific is the observed effect?
- Is there a pharmacological basis for the suspected drug effect?

Often, there is insufficient data to provide conclusive answers to these questions. Where relevant data are available, more often than not this relates to the effects on male sexual functioning. The relationship between therapeutic medication, ill-health and sexual functioning is a complex one. For example, the use of anti-depressants, especially those with a pronounced serotonergic effect, is associated with sexual side-effects, although the precise incidence of these deleterious side-effects is unknown (Segraves, 1998). Depression itself, however, is associated with a loss of sexual interest (Hawton, 1985) and the use of anti-depressants may help ameliorate this by elevating mood.

Certain drugs with anti-androgenic properties are used therapeutically for the treatment of certain cancers. The synthetic gonadotropin-releasing hormone (GnRH) analogue Buserelin, which is used in palliative treatment of advanced prostatic cancer and advanced male breast cancer, often results in loss of sexual desire and impairment of erections (Murphy, 1998). Some anti-androgen drugs, such as cyproterone acetate, have also been used in the treatment of male hypersexuality. However, the most commonly encountered drugs with anti-androgenic properties are cimetidine, metoclopramide and digoxin. Although these drugs are not used as anti-androgens, their effect on the endocrine system is a side-effect (Murphy, 1998). The 'non-sexual' side-effects of certain therapeutic drugs, for fatigue, nausea, vomiting and diarrhoea for example, may alter an individual's interest in sex. Sometimes it is the concomitant changes in body image, be it alopecia caused by cytotoxic chemotherapy, skin and weight changes associated with corticosteroids or the presence of indwelling catheters through which treatments can be administered, that have an adverse effect upon sexual relationships.

When trying to appraise whether a persisting alteration in sexual response is a possible drug side-effect, practitioners also need to be aware that a number of non-prescription medications and 'recreational' drugs may also interfere with sexual functioning. Tomlinson (1998) notes that many 'cold cures' and 'over the counter' hypnotics contain anti-cholinergic agents, such as diphenhydramine. Alcohol may initially enhance sexual expression through relaxation or disinhibition, but when consumed in excess is associated with erectile dysfunction, with 50–80% of male alcoholics experiencing erectile dysfunction (Gregoire, 1999a). Cigarette smoking is also associated epidemiologically with erectile dysfunction. This may be due to its association with vascular disease, however, the rapid restoration of erectile function following the cessation of smoking reported by some people points possibly to a more direct effect of nicotine on sexual functioning (Bancroft, 1989). Murphy (1998) reports that users of Ecstasy (3,4-methylenedioxymethamphetamine) report enhancement of the sensuous aspects of sex, but inhibition of orgasm and ejaculation. The heavy or prolonged use of marijuana, opiates and many other 'recreational' drugs is associated with deleterious effects on sexual response.

Responses to illness and disability

Illness and disability may alter sexual expression through the effects that they have on an individual's body image, self-concept, self-esteem and social roles (Webb, 1985). Any alteration in the way individuals view themselves is often reflected and reinforced by the reactions of other people, and can cause emotional and sexual disturbance. This in turn may further alter an individual's perception of self and the responses he or she receives from others, thereby perpetuating emotional and sexual problems. Possible psychological responses to illness or disability that may alter sexual response in this way include the following.

Anticipatory failure and fear of harm or pain

Although the effects of surgery and illness on sexual function are often transient, they may become permanent if failure is anticipated or one aspect of sexual response remains impaired (Hawton, 1985). Concern about possible 'failure to perform' sometimes leads to the avoidance of sexual activity, as does fear of causing harm or pain. Patients who have had heart attacks may especially fear provoking further attacks, and patients who have undergone surgery, especially gynaecological or urological, may desist unnecessarily from sexual activity for fear of causing damage. Providing the patient with permission to be sexually active following illness, surgery or other forms of treatment may be achieved with a simple enquiry as to how sex is following surgery or treatment. Such a question may also elicit any underlying anxieties or concerns.

Altered body image

Changes to body image may alter self-concept, threaten self-esteem and thereby affect an individual's sense of his or her attractiveness to others. Altered body image may occur as a result of illness, trauma, surgery and treatments such as radiotherapy and chemotherapy. It is not only changes to body shape that lead to an altered body image but also changes in bodily functions, such as immobility, incontinence, sensory impairment and sexual dysfunction. Although cancers and treatments that alter the physical structure of the genitals and breasts might be expected to have psychosexual sequealae secondary to changes in body image, a number of studies indicate that between a third and quarter of patients with a variety of cancers report changes in sexual self-concept and sexual interest (Maguire and Parkes, 1998).

Loss

There are numerous losses which ill-health and injury can bring, and loss may generate emotional responses such as anxiety or depression which, in turn, result in further losses (Parkes and Markus, 1998). Loss not only disturbs one's sense of self (and therefore one's sexuality) but can make it difficult to maintain relationships as the pain associated with loss often means that 'the focus of feelings turns to the self and there is a retreat from relationships with others' (Clifford, 2000a, p. 86). Clifford states that such feelings of loss in patients require acknowledgement rather than reassurance from practitioners and considers that where it is clear to clinicians that loss of whatever kind is inevitable, there is a responsibility to prepare the patient for this. This would include alerting patients to any possible effect on sexual functioning before elective surgery or other courses of treatment.

Reactions of partners

Partners too may also worry about the effect of ill-health and treatment on the patient's sexual functioning or may believe that after treatment sexual activity will be impossible or inadvisable if there is the possibility of causing pain or doing harm. Sexual problems are more likely to occur if a couple has difficulty discussing their sexual relationship (Hawton, 1985), although guilt arising from a conflict between sexual desire and concerns about a partner's physical health may also lead to the avoidance of sexual activity and consequent resentment and relationship difficulties. Altschuler (1997) observes that ill-health often disturbs the equilibrium of personal relationships, altering how needs for intimacy and distance are experienced, expressed and managed. In chronic illness or disability, changes in a couple's sexual relationship may occur as a consequence of altered roles within the couple relationship. This is perhaps most obvious when one partner becomes the other's 'carer' (Webster and Heath, 2001). Sexual problems are also more likely to occur if sexual difficulties existed in a relationship prior to the changes brought about by illness or disability (Hawton, 1985).

The effects of ageing on sexual response

Although sexual interest and activity tend to decline in later life, many older people continue to have an active and enjoyable sex life. Spence (1991) observes that patterns of sexual activity in old age tend to reflect a person's sexual behaviour in earlier years. Read (1999) suggests that people who have been sexually active on a frequent basis throughout their lives tend to show a lower rate of decline in sexual activity than those who have been less sexually active. Read (1999) also reminds practitioners that the range of sexual interests and preferences in older people is just as wide as that found in younger people. Spence (1991) writes that although physiological changes in sexual responding occur with age, these are insufficient to explain the decrease in sexual interest and activity found among many older people. The effects of these normal physiological changes on sexual response are listed in Table 4.2 and are discussed in greater detail by Spence (1991), Gibson (1992) and Trudel et al. (2000).

Gibson (1992) concludes that, in general, women alter less than men physiologically with ageing except for the menopause which affects the level of the sex steroids that are available, and this varies very greatly between individuals.

Table 4.2: Ageing and changes in sexual response

The female sexual response:
    more stimulation required for vaginal lubrication and distension to occur
    less obvious changes in the labia majora and minora which make penetration easier
    minor anatomical changes in the erect clitoris similar to those of the penis
    altered and shortened orgasm – either fewer reflex uterine contractions on orgasm or a
    spasm of the uterus rather than a rhythmic contraction
    uncertainty exists about the effects of ageing on the capacity to experience multiple
    orgasms
The male sexual response:
    more stimulation required for the penis to become erect
    the erect penis may not be as elevated or as firm as it was previously
    greater time taken for ejaculation to occur
    greater variability in terms of ejaculatory response
    less semen ejaculated with considerably less force
    longer 'refractory period' following ejaculation

The menopause

The meaning and significance of the 'change of life' vary greatly between women and their partners, making it difficult to generalize about the nature of the difficulties experienced at this stage of life. Denman (1995) observes that whilst some women are devastated by the loss of their fertility, others are often very pleased to be relieved of the possibility of becoming pregnant. Although in some societies the climacteric and cessation of childbearing brings new-found freedoms, in Western societies ageing women may feel they are becoming undesirable and 'invisible' to current or potential sexual partners. Denman (1995) notes that if a woman's pre-existing sexual relationship has been poor, it is unlikely to improve at this stage. Sexual difficulties, including a decline in sexual desire, are often associated with menopausal status, although other factors such as stress, ill-health and relationship problems in addition to the menopause may contribute to such difficulties.

Denman (1995) suggests that there are, however, a number of specific problems that are directly related to the menopause. The first of these she describes as the 'domino effect'. Vasomotor symptoms experienced by many women during the menopause, such as night sweats and hot flushes, not only cause embarrassment, loss of confidence and lowered mood for some women but may also lead to insomnia and consequently fatigue. This in turn may adversely affect sexual desire. Denman (1995) notes that relief of vasomotor symptoms by use of hormone replacement therapy (HRT) may also ameliorate any secondary difficulties. The second problem Denman (1995) describes is the consequence of atrophic symptoms that are secondary to lower levels of circulating oestrogen. As ovarian function declines, levels of oestrogen also diminish, causing a thinning of the epithelium of the vulva and vagina, and reduced lubrication during sexual intercourse. Often this results in vulvo-vaginal soreness, irritation and dyspareunia. The expectation of painful sexual intercourse may, in turn, reduce sexual interest and lead to the avoidance of sexual activity. Although atrophic symptoms may be resolved with appropriate use of systemic HRT or topical oestrogen in the form of pessaries or cream, some women still retain a fear or expectation of pain associated with sexual intercourse which leads to an involuntary contraction of vaginal muscles when penetration is attempted. This vaginismus leads to pain thereby reinforcing the perception that 'something is still wrong inside'. Denman (1995) suggests that a therapeutic genital examination and explanation may help to break this vicious circle of pain, fear and vaginismus.

A 'male menopause'?

The concept of a 'male menopause' is still the subject of considerable debate (see Gould et al., 2000). The term is generally deemed inappropriate as it erroneously implies a sudden drop in sex hormones similar to that of peri-menopausal women. It is recognized that, with normal ageing, testosterone levels do decline gradually in men, although there is considerable variability between individuals and a broad range in age-related values. Some of the symptoms associated with lowered levels of testosterone include:

- Vasomotor symptoms.
- Mood changes.
- Decreased sexual interest.
- Erectile problems.
- Fatigue.
- Difficulties associated with memory and concentration.

Some commentators have advocated the use of 'androgen replacement therapy' in elderly men experiencing such symptoms. Gould and Petty (in Gould et al., 2000) cite various studies which suggest that testosterone replacement may help ameliorate vasomotor disturbances and night sweats, improve energy levels and reduce tiredness, improve sexual interest and help with erectile difficulties in a sizable proportion of elderly men experiencing such problems. However, in the same article Jacobs (Gould et al., 2000) writes that the role of testosterone with regard to sexual activity in elderly men is still not well-defined and cites research which suggests that circulating concentrations of testosterone in older men are usually well above those required for a normal sexual response. Reviewing the available research, Jacobs (in Gould et al., 2000) concludes that the case for androgen replacement therapy in elderly men who do not have biochemically indicated testosterone deficiency (hypogonadism) has yet to be proven.

Health and psychosocial influences

Because of the greater probability (although not inevitability) of underlying health-related problems, it is essential that practitioners encountering older patients who present with a persisting impairment of sexual function, recommend that they attend for appropriate medical assessment and investigation. It is also important to remember that any alteration in sexual interest or response reported by patients may also be the consequence of sexual dysfunction in their partners that is secondary to ill-health or side-effects of prescribed medications. In addition to ill-health and possible iatrogenic causes of altered sexual function, a number of psychosocial influences may affect sexual responding either directly or through their effect on an individual's self-concept, self-esteem and social roles, including:

- Changes in living arrangements.
- Lack of suitable partners.
- Retirement.
- Loss of a long-term partner.

Cosmetic changes in physical appearance which accompany ageing may also have a strong influence on a person's sexual identity and sexual relationships in a society which equates sexual attractiveness with signs of youth (Grigg, 1999; Trudel et al., 2000). Spence (1991) observes that although many older people fear that their partner will no longer find them physically attractive, for the majority of couples this fear is unfounded. However, concern about no longer being sexually attractive may be reinforced by a lack of communication or misattributing changes in the sexual interest shown by one's partner. Clifford (2000a) notes that there is a tendency to equate lack of sexual desire with lack of affection and to attribute a partner's lack of sexual interest to one's self – *'I'm no longer physically attractive'* – rather than consider other possible explanations, such as incipient ill-heath, depression or iatrogenesis. A vicious circle of perceived rejection, lowered self-esteem and altered sexual response may quickly become established (Read, 1999).

The death of a long-term partner is a source of extreme stress and disturbance for most people and losses which are 'hidden' or concealed, may cause particular distress and difficulties (*see* Parkes, 1998). As Rutter (2000a) notes:

> One of the most difficult experiences of grief is that following secret love, e.g. in a gay relationship that has not been socially recognized, or in an extra-marital relationship when the couple is unable to spend their final days together. (Rutter, 2000a, p. 205)

For some people, however, the death of a partner may be associated with enormous relief, especially if it brings to an end a long and painful terminal illness or the relationship had been a very difficult one. Some people may experience a considerable amount of guilt for experiencing such relief, others will not. Parkes (1998) suggests that:

> Time spent in creating the secure place in which people feel safe enough to talk about the unsafe thoughts and feelings that they are experiencing is likely to prevent further problems and may well save time in the long run. (Parkes, 1998, p. 87)

After experiencing the loss of a long term partner, sexual pleasure, be it in the form of masturbation or in response to the stimulus provided by another person, may generate considerable anxiety and a sense of guilt in some people. This, in turn, may lead to psychosexual difficulties that either disrupt the formation of new relationships, or cause an individual to eschew completely any opportunity to gain the emotional support and affection that he or she needs.

Kaplan (1974) writes that the majority of complaints concerning sexuality and ageing are the consequence of a lack of knowledge of normal physiological changes associated with increasing age and an inability to communicate needs and preferences. Although it would be wrong to equate sexual self-concept entirely with sexual function, it is necessary to recognize how changes in sexual function may adversely affect a person's sexual identity and vice versa. Similarly, it would be wrong to assume that the sexual aspect of a relationship is of great significance for all older people, or couples, but also equally wrong to equate ageing with inevitable sexual decrepitude and abstinence. The social expectation that equates senescence with asexuality often inhibits the communication that is necessary to resolve such difficulties. Patients often feel too embarrassed to ask for outside help with such problems and often feel disinclined to talk directly about changes in sexual feelings with their partners. As Heath (2001) writes:

> Two pervasive inhibitors of older people's sexuality in contemporary Western society are the myth that sexual interest is inappropriate to feel and the stereotype that its expression is unwelcome. (Health, 2001, p. 133)

Psychological and interpersonal aspects of sexual problems

The psychosocial factors associated with sexual problems are often divided into predisposing factors, precipitants and maintaining factors (Hawton, 1985; Daines and Perrett, 2000). Spence (1991) notes, however, that although such a classification of psychosocial factors is appealing, it is often very difficult in practice to determine whether a factor is a precipitating event or is helping to maintain a change in sexual response.

Predisposing factors

Predisposing factors are those previous experiences that make people more susceptible to sexual difficulties which often do not emerge until much later in their lives. Examples of predisposing factors include:

- Early patterns of socialization.
- Inadequate sexual information and 'sexual myths'.
- Traumatic early sexual experiences, such as childhood sexual abuse.

Hawton (1985) suggests that children's experience of their family attitudes towards sexuality and personal relationships is likely to have a profound effect on their psychosexual development. Such familial attitudes may be expressed both overtly and covertly. The relationship between the experience of childhood sexual abuse and sexual difficulties later in life is considered in Chapter 9. Spence (1991) suggests that with regard to sex and sexuality, people tend to hold beliefs and attitudes concerning a wide range of issues including:

- What sexual activities are deemed 'normal', pleasurable and in what situations such activities are acceptable.
- The roles during sexual activity (who does what to whom – when, where and why).
- What constitutes 'good sex'.

Precipitants

'Precipitants' are events which trigger a change in sexual interest or response. These are the causal factors that patients are most likely to be aware of. Possible precipitants include:

- Childbirth and parenthood.
- Altered sexual response in a partner.
- Relationship difficulties, including infidelity.
- Random failure.
- Reaction to ill-health.
- Ageing.
- Depression or anxiety.
- Sexual assault or rape.
- Bereavement.

The term 'random failure' in the above list refers to 'one-off' failure of sexual response that can sometimes precipitate a sexual dysfunction because of the psychological sequelae of such an episode. The partner's response to the occurrence of a sexual difficulty seems particularly important in determining whether such difficulties are likely to recur. Conversely, the reciprocal nature of sexual interaction means that any alteration in one partner's sexual response may also bring changes in the other partner's sexual functioning.

Maintaining factors

Alteration in sexual response tends only to become problematic if it persists, and the factors that perpetuate sexual difficulties are known as 'maintaining factors'. Potential maintaining factors:

- Avoidance of sexual activity
- Performance anxiety and anticipation of failure.
- Guilt.

- Relationship difficulties, including poor communication between partners.
- Impaired self-image.
- Inadequate information.
- Fear of intimacy.
- Loss of attraction between partners.
- Poor problem-solving skills.
- Psychiatric illness.
- Social and situational factors, such as lack of privacy, stress at work or prejudice.

Many commentators have suggested that anxiety plays a major role in the inhibition of sexual interest, sexual arousal and orgasm, and may act as a predisposing factor, precipitating and maintaining factor. Daines and Perrett (2000) note, for example, that a high level of generalized anxiety might make an individual more vulnerable to sexual difficulties and that a period of acute anxiety or stress may trigger a sexual problem. Anxiety may also act as a maintaining factor for a sexual problem through the processes of performance anxiety, anticipatory failure and 'spectatoring'. Spectatoring is a term used to describe a situation where an individual's mind is focused on his or her sexual performance to the exclusion of almost everything else. Research suggests that anxiety generated by explicit or implicit demands for sexual performance, inhibits sexual arousal in those experiencing sexual problems but facilitates it in those who are not experiencing such problems. Thus, the relationship between anxiety and sexual response is a complex one, and it would appear that sexual dysfunction occurs as a consequence of the interaction of cognitive processes and anxiety (Barlow, 1986).

Relationship difficulties and sexual problems

Any change in sexual interest or response must always be evaluated in terms of the relationships in which it manifests (Watson and Davies, 1997). In one study of 200 couples referred to a psychosexual problems clinic, one-third had significant marital and relationship problems (Catalan et al., 1990). Daines and Perrett (2000) note three relationship factors that may contribute to sexual problems. These are:

- Differences of sexual interest.
- Difficulties in communicating about sex.

- General relationship difficulties causing a sexual problem.

Daines and Perrett (2000) argue that difference of interest in sex is primarily a relational problem since it might not occur with a different partner who has a similar level of sexual interest. Difficulties communicating about sex may be part of a more general communication problem, although often many couples cannot communicate about sex despite communicating well about other issues. It is common for couples to assume that they know each other's sexual needs, likes and dislikes, and many couples deem talking about sexual practices to be abnormal or undesirable. Consequently, many people put up with sexual practices that they do not enjoy, or that have become boring to them (Daines and Perrett, 2000).

Most relationship problems occur as a result of difficulties relating to communication, conflict and commitment (Watson and Davies, 1997). Daines and Perrett (2000) suggest that in order to engage in a sexual relationship, most people need to be able to feel vulnerable without feeling unsafe and that this is not possible if significant degrees of resentment, anger or hostility are present in a relationship. Conversely, a relationship problem can be secondary to a sexual problem as 'it is difficult for any relationship to contain a sexual problem for a long time without it affecting other areas of the relationship' (Daines and Perrett, 2000, p. 36).

Implications for nursing practice

Recognizing and responding to psychosexual anxieties and distress are examples of secondary preventative sexual health care in that these interventions may help patients to avoid more serious or intractable sexual and relationship difficulties and avert further distress. An awareness of the potential changes that ill-health, disability and treatment may bring to a patient's self concept, sexual expression, function and satisfaction can enable practitioners to provide a degree of primary preventative sexual health care to many of their patients. Preparing patients for the sexual changes that may occur following illness, treatment, or 'life events', may help diminish, if not avert, subsequent psychosexual concerns. Such preparation requires practitioners not only to give patients the opportunity and 'permission' to express any concerns about the impact of illness and treatment on their sexual expression or relationships but also to provide specific information about the potential sexual side-effects of treatment; the behavioural responses that may compound any sexual difficulties (e.g.

avoidance of sexual activity, non-communication between partners); and when, after acute illness or treatment, sexual activity can be safely resumed (Hawton, 1985).

The second element of preventative psychosexual care is the prompt identification of any changes in sexual interest, function or satisfaction that may follow medical or surgical treatment. This can be done with the judicious and sensitive use of 'cue' questions (*see* Chapter 3) or by using a more formal assessment protocol, such as the ALARM model proposed by Andersen (1990). ALARM is an acronym for:

- Activity: What are the patient's normal levels of interest in sex, modes of sexual expression and types of sexual relationships?
- Libido: Have there been any changes in the patient's level of sexual interest, and what are the significance and importance of any such changes for the patient? Is the patient satisfied with the current situation?
- Arousal: Does the patient identify any specific changes in sexual function and if so, have these changes led to any emotional disturbance or disruption of relationships?
- Resolution: Is the experience (or not) of orgasm satisfactory for the patient? Does the patient experience any problems with pain or discomfort?
- Medical history: What is the patient's past medical history? Is the patient currently taking any medication that may impair sexual interest or response? Are there any underlying physical issues that still need to be explored?

Kelly (2001, p. 204) states that 'this format for approaching sexual assessment may be of practical use in busy settings and provides a structure within which sensitive questions can be phrased'.

The third aspect of preventative psychosexual care is helping patients with sexual adjustment after irreparable body changes or in response to progressive debility. Nursing intervention at this level usually involves making specific suggestions designed to:

- Ameliorate mechanical problems.
- Relieve pain and discomfort.
- Identify ways of optimizing residual sexual function.
- Adjust sexual activities to limitations placed on patient's ability for physical exertion.

This level of nursing practice requires, among other things, a detailed knowledge of the impact of illness and disability upon sexual expression, and consequently, is usually provided by specialist practitioners (*see* Chapter 1). When caring for patients with underlying medical conditions or disabilities who report sexual difficulties, it is important for practitioners not to presume that the patient's sexual problems are causally related to their medical condition or disability. As Riley and Riley (1988, p. 271) note: 'Patients with medical disease can develop sexual difficulties for all the same reasons as a physically fit person, the medical disease being a concurrent but unrelated problem.'

Key points of Chapter 4

- Sexual activity is a psychosomatic event. Any alteration in sexual interest or sexual response is usually the result of a combination of physical, psychological and interpersonal factors.
- A number of physical factors may alter sexual interest and sexual function. These include endocrine, neurological and cardiovascular conditions; trauma; and iatrogenic factors such as the side-effects of certain prescribed treatments, and damage caused by certain types of surgery.
- The reactions of patients and their partners to ill-health, treatment and the consequences of these, may also result in changes in sexual interest and response.
- A number of drugs that are used recreationally, such as alcohol and nicotine, may also impair sexual response.
- Physiological changes in sexual responding also occur with age, although these are generally insufficient to explain the decrease in sexual interest and activity observed in many older people.
- Psychosocial factors contributing to changes in sexual interest or response are conventionally divided into predisposing, precipitating and maintaining factors. In practice, this division of psychosocial factors is harder to discern.
- Alterations in sexual interest, response or satisfaction need to be evaluated in the context of the relationships in which they occur.
- How the implications of physical illness, surgery and other forms of treatment are dealt with by practitioners can determine a patient's subsequent sexual adjustment.

Key reading

Kelly, D. (2001) Sexuality and people with acute illness. In: Health, H., White, I. (eds). *The Challenge of Sexuality in Health Care*. London: Blackwell Science.

Gill, M. (2001) Interaction of physical and psychological factors. In: Skrine, R., Montford, H. (eds). *Psychosexual Medicine: An Introduction* (second edition). London: Arnold.

CHAPTER 5

Sexual dysfunction

Introduction

In a recent survey of a non-clinical sample of the population carried out in the UK, two-fifths of female and a third of male respondents reported having a current sexual problem. The most common male problems were erectile dysfunction and premature ejaculation, and the most common female problems were vaginal dryness and infrequency of orgasm. Of those who reported having a sexual problem, 52% indicated they would like to receive professional help for their problem, although only one in ten had received any such help (Dunn, et al., 1998). The purpose of this chapter is to provide practitioners with an overview of sexual dysfunctions that describes both the possible origins and management of this type of sexual difficulty. The assessment and treatment of sexual dysfunctions is outside both the remit and expertise of all but suitably trained and supervised practitioners. Guidance is therefore given concerning the referral of such patients, and the sources of specialist help that may be available to them.

Sexual dysfunction

Hawton (1985, p. 30) offers what he terms a working definition of sexual dysfunction as 'the persistent impairment of normal patterns of sexual interest or response'. Hawton (1985) acknowledges, however, that this definition has two particular problems. First, what is 'normal' is perhaps difficult to describe given that the range of sexual interest and sexual activities in humans is so broad. It is not only the quantity and type of sexual activity which vary greatly between individuals but also the importance (or not) and meanings attached to such activities. Hawton

Table 5.1: Classification of sexual problems

Aspect of sexual response	Female	Male
Desire	Impaired sexual desire	Impaired sexual desire
Arousal	Impaired sexual arousal	Erectile dysfunction
Orgasm	Orgasmic dysfunction	Premature ejaculation
		Delayed/absent ejaculation
Other	Dyspareunia	Dyspareunia
	Vaginismus	
	Sexual phobia	Sexual phobia

(1985) notes that any judgement concerning whether or not an individual has a sexual dysfunction that requires treatment, should depend on whether a person feels that there is a problem.

The American Psychiatric Association's fourth edition of its *Diagnostic and Statistical Manual of Mental Disorder* (DSM-IV) (APA, 1995) and the World Health Organization's *International Classification of Diseases* (ICD-10) (WHO, 1992) each have a classification system and diagnostic criteria for sexual dysfunction. Generally, a 'persistent' impairment of sexual interest or response is taken to mean that which has persisted for longer than six months. However, the diagnostic categories described in both the ICD-10 and DSM-IV do not always reflect the realities of sexual dysfunction presented by patients in clinical settings (Gregoire, 1999a). Hawton (1985) provides a classification system, which encompasses disturbances of both sexual interest and sexual function (Table 5.1); this is commonly utilized by many clinicians working in the area of sexual dysfunction.

Each of the sexual difficulties listed in Table 5.1 may also be sub-typed according to whether they are *primary* or *secondary* problems. A primary sexual problem is one that has been present since first sexual activity, whereas a secondary sexual problem is one that has developed following a period of unproblematic sexual activity. Sexual problems may also be classified according to whether they are *total* or *situational*. A total problem is one that is present all the time, whereas a situational problem occurs only under certain circumstances or in certain situations (Masters and Johnson, 1970). Additionally, sexual problems are often classified according to whether they are deemed to be physical or psychological in origin, or are the result of a combination of psychological and physical factors.

Impaired sexual interest

Also referred to as 'impaired sexual desire' and 'hypoactive sexual desire disorder' in other classification systems, or 'loss of libido' is, according to Hawton (1985) the most common problem among women seen in sexual dysfunction clinics. Hawton (1985) suggests that men may be more likely to seek help for 'performance disorders' such as erectile problems, although these may be the result of reduced sexual interest. The term 'impaired sexual interest' may be used to describe a wide range of difficulties. It may be used to refer to a lack of any spontaneous interest in sex in a person who remains responsive to a partner's sexual approaches. It may also refer to situations when initial sexual interest is lost once sexual activity commences. It can also refer to a total lack of any interest in sex and aversion to the sexual approaches of partners.

Hawton (1985) suggests that negative experiences in early life are often important aetiological factors in women with primary impairment of sexual interest, whereas relationship difficulties or precipitants such as childbirth are often implicated in secondary impairment of sexual interest. Conditions and drugs that cause hyperprolactinaemia may also have a direct effect on reducing a woman's sex drive, as may androgen deficiency syndrome after hysterectomy and bilateral salpingo-oophorectomy, or chemotherapy for cancer (Butcher, 1999). Hawton (1985) suggests that certain myths and stereotypes about male sexuality – that men are always interested in sex and ready to 'perform' – may make it particularly difficult for men to acknowledge any absence or reduction in sexual interest. When impaired interest in sex is a primary problem in men, the possibility of a physical cause, such as an endocrine disturbance, needs to be considered. Impaired sexual interest in both men and women may be the consequence of changes in personal relationships, loss, depression or any protracted illness or disability.

Impaired sexual arousal

This refers to a failure of the physiological responses, such as vaginal lubrication and swelling, and the lack of sensations an individual usually associates with sexual excitement. Daines and Perrett (2000) suggest that the absence of sexual excitement is usually psychological in origin and that a lack of sexual arousal is often a defence against feeling sexual in order to avoid guilt or other negative feelings. Hormonal changes following childbirth and the menopause may impair the normal vaginal response to sexual stimulation, as may medical conditions such as coronary heart disease and hypertension, where vaginal or clitoral blood flow is diminished (Berman and Berman, 2001).

Erectile dysfunction

This is common male problem as erectile response is very vulnerable to disruption caused by physical disorders (especially those of the neurological, endocrine and cardiovascular systems), the side-effects of many medications and 'recreational' drugs, such as alcohol and nicotine, and psychological factors, such as anxiety. The range of problems which constitute an erectile dysfunction is considerable. Primary total erectile dysfunction is relatively rare and usually has its origin in organic factors. A physical cause is also more likely when a man can obtain partial erections. Erectile dysfunction where a man can obtain erections on his own but not with his partner or cannot sustain his erection when sexual activity commences is usually psychological in origin and/or maintenance (Hawton, 1985).

Orgasmic dysfunction

This term is used to describe difficulty, delay or absence of orgasm in women. It is important to note that many women enjoy sexual activity without reaching orgasm and that the absence of orgasm in such circumstances is not necessarily problematic. Primary total orgasmic dysfunction is relatively common, although Hawton (1985) notes that the number of women presenting for help with this problem seems to be declining and suggests that this might be the result of the increasing number of articles in popular magazines about masturbation and how to attain an orgasm and the greater availability of self-help books. Daines and Perrett (2000), however, observe that the increasing emphasis in society placed on becoming orgasmic may have a negative effect on some women, making it difficult for them to attend to their own needs. Secondary orgasmic dysfunction, that is, difficulties associated with attaining an orgasm in women who have previously been orgasmic, may occur for physical, psychological or interpersonal reasons. Hypopituitarism, multiple sclerosis, malignant disease, the side-effects of certain medications, damage to pelvic nerves during surgery and hormone deficiencies may all contribute to secondary orgasmic dysfunction (Berman and Berman, 2001; Vanhegan, 2001). Secondary orgasmic dysfunction may also occur because of a lack of sexual interest following a trauma, such as rape or termination of pregnancy, or as a consequence of difficulties in a woman's relationship with her partner.

Premature ejaculation

Premature ejaculation is difficult to define satisfactorily, but refers to a situation where the timing of ejaculation leads to dissatisfaction for a man or his partner. This dissatisfaction may, in part, be the result of unrealistic expectations derived from a number of sexual myths and misconceptions (Baker and deSilva, 1988). Rapid ejaculation is common in young men having their first sexual encounter, but subsequently most men develop a certain control over their speed of ejaculation. Premature ejaculation is usually a primary problem and there is often a history of rapid masturbation, sometimes associated with guilt, or early sexual experiences in uncomfortable or anxiety-producing situations (Daines and Perrett, 2000; Whitmore, 2001). The reaction of a man's partner to his rapid ejaculation is also crucial, as responses of anger or condemnation may compound the problem. Premature ejaculation can also be both a cause of, and a response to, sexual problems in partners such as painful intercourse resulting from lack of sexual arousal (Daines and Perrett, 2000).

Hawton (1985) observes that for many young men the brief refractory period following first ejaculation often compensates for premature ejaculation in that they are able to sustain sex for longer prior to ejaculating a second time. As the refractory period subsequently lengthens with ageing, premature ejaculation may become problematic. Secondary premature ejaculation sometimes develops at times of stress or following a period of sexual abstinence. It may also precede erectile dysfunction caused by other factors.

Delayed ejaculation

This is sometimes referred to as 'retarded ejaculation'. Delayed ejaculation is a relatively uncommon complaint but includes a range of problems, such as a complete inability to ejaculate under any circumstances, the ability to ejaculate with masturbation but not in the presence of a sexual partner, and ejaculation that occurs only after what is perceived to be an excessively long period of time and sexual stimulation. Several types of medication can interfere with ejaculation and Hawton (1985) suggests that a total failure of ejaculation is likely to have a physical cause. A number of psychological factors, some of them unconscious, may also lead to delayed ejaculation, including the effects of restrictive upbringing, anxiety, anger, an inabililty to 'let go' emotionally, difficulties with emotional intimacy, and the fear or becoming a father (Whitmore, 2001).

Vaginismus

Vaginismus is defined by Basson et al. (2000, p. 890) as 'the recurrent or persistent involuntary spasm of the musculature of the outer third of the vagina that interferes with vaginal penetration, which causes personal distress'. Vaginismus is usually a primary dysfunction, although it may develop as a secondary problem following vaginal trauma or as a consequence of recurrent vaginal infection (Hawton, 1985). Secondary vaginismus may also occur as a result of relationship and emotional difficulties, after sexual abuse or assault, or when pregnancy is feared.

Both Hawton (1985) and Daines and Perrett (2000) suggest that some women who present with vaginismus as a primary dysfunction may have a specific phobia about vaginal penetration that is reflected in difficulties in the use of tampons, extreme fears about childbirth or distorted ideas about the size and/or structure of the vagina. As many women with vaginismus enjoy other forms of sexual activity, and are often sexually responsive to manual or oral stimulation, a dislike of penetrative sex is not necessarily an indication of a sexual problem but may be an expression of a woman's sexual preferences (Daines and Perrett, 2000, p. 30).

Dyspareunia

This refers to pain during sexual intercourse. Pain located at the entrance of the vagina may be the result of lack of adequate sexual arousal, mild vaginismus, a Bartholin's cyst or vulvo-vaginal infection. Pain that occurs 'deep' in the vagina often has a physical cause, such a vaginal infection, pelvic infection, cervical or ovarian pathology and endometriosis. Sometimes, however, deep dyspareunia is the consequence of impaired sexual arousal when expansion of the inner vagina and elevation of the uterus do not occur (Hawton, 1985). Dyspareunia is often reported during pregnancy and may be the consequence of a variety of physical, psychological and interpersonal factors (Aston, 2001). Although there are a number of physical causes of dyspareunia, it may also occur as a result of fears about infections or pregnancy, anger or resentment in a current relationship, or unresolved feelings about previous abuse, or difficulties encountered in giving birth or bereavement (Davis, 2001).

Pain associated with sexual activity may occur also for some men. Causes of such pain include problems with the foreskin, a tear in the frenulum and infection involving the urethra, seminal vesicles, prostate gland or bladder. Hawton (1985) also notes that some men experience hyperaesthesia of the glans penis after ejaculation that causes the glans to

be very painful if touched. Daines and Perrett (2000) suggest that
sometimes men experience pain associated with sexual activity which has a
psychological origin. They also note there are a significant number of men
for whom no identifiable cause for their pain can be found.

Sexual phobia

Sometimes called 'sexual aversion disorder', sexual phobia may occur as
an isolated problem or be associated with other dysfunctions, such as
impaired sexual interest, erectile dysfunction, impaired sexual arousal or
vaginismus. Daines and Perrett (2000) suggest that sexual phobias are a
defence against anxiety-causing situations, such as touch or intimacy,
consequently they can be very specific, for example an aversion to
touching a partner's genitals, or may cause anxiety that militates against
any form of sexual contact.

The limitations of conventional classification systems

Most current classification systems of sexual dysfunctions give the
impression that each dysfunction is a discrete entity. In clinical practice,
co-morbidity of sexual dysfunction occurs frequently (Rosen and Leiblum,
1995). Often, impaired sexual interest is concurrent with alteration in
sexual function, although the former, being less 'observable' and therefore
'quantifiable', is less likely to be the presenting problem. Co-morbidity of
sexual dysfunctions may not only occur in an individual but may also occur
in a couple. Gregoire (1999a) observes that in up to a third of partners of
individuals with sexual problems also have a sexual dysfunction.

   Furthermore, each category of sexual dysfunction contains a wide
spectrum of variations in sexual response which may vary in both severity
and frequency (Gregoire, 1999a). Rosen and Leiblum (1995) also observe
that current classification systems are based on a dichotomous view of
sexual health as being either functional or dysfunction, whereas sexual
functioning might better be represented on a continuum of individual or
interpersonal satisfaction.

   In addition to dichotomizing sexual health into functional and
dysfunctional, sexual problems in most classification systems are often
defined in terms of the disruption caused to penile–vaginal intercourse.
The notion of a 'sexual problem' is too often underpinned by a
psychosexual perspective that 'all too often assumes "sex" to be

heterosexual, penile–vaginal intercourse leading to orgasm – though this form of sexual activity may be undesirable, unavailable or impossible for many people' (Savage, 1987, p. 50). This is slowly changing. In their proposed new classification system for female dysfunction, Basson et al. (2000, p. 890) include a category of 'non-coital sexual pain disorder' which they define as 'recurrent or persistent genital pain induced by noncoital sexual stimulation'. Basson and colleagues state that they included this category in their proposed classification system because a significant number of women experience pain during non-coital forms of sexual stimulation and as recognition 'that sexual activity for women need not necessarily involve penile vaginal intercourse and the category of sexual pain disorder may apply to nonheterosexual women engaging in alternative sexual behaviours' (Basson et al., 2000, p. 891). Similarly, Rosser et al. (1998) propose that 'anodyspareunia' (persistent or recurrent severe pain associated with receptive anal sex) be included as a sexual pain disorder. This is important given that approximately a third of heterosexual couples are thought to use anal sex as an occasional method of sexual expression (with about 10% using it as the preferred or regular method) and that up to two-thirds of gay men practise anal sex as a regular sexual activity (Bell, 1999).

Finally, Crowe (1998) makes the point that the two most widely used diagnostic manuals for sexual problems – the ICD-10 and the DSM-IV – still retain an implicit assumption that a sexual problem 'belongs' to only one person, thereby neglecting the relationship aspects of sexual difficulties.

The response of the nurse

Practitioners will on occasions encounter patients whose psychosexual anxiety and distress is the consequence of a persistent alteration in their normal sexual function. Faced with distress in such circumstances, practitioners may feel they need to generate solutions to patients' problems. Selby (2000) offers the following caution to practitioners:

> The need to find a solution to your patient's anxieties could mean that you start advising on techniques in sexual nursing for which you have not trained. The work of Masters and Johnson (1970) and their techniques (a behaviourist therapy) are frequently quoted and offered by some nurses to their patients because it is seen to be constructive and better than nothing. This is not good practice, as all recognized therapies require training, practice and supervision. (Selby, 2000, p. 88)

Psychosexual awareness is about recognizing and responding to the sexual anxieties and distress of patients; it is not intended to be a 'treatment' for sexual dysfunctions. The recognition of sexual anxiety and distress may help some patients who are experiencing such problems, but psychosexual nursing is not a form of psychosexual therapy. Most patients with sexual dysfunction will require referral for specialist assessment and help. Although they are not providers of psychosexual therapy it is important that practitioners are able to recognize when referral is appropriate and discuss with patients what such treatment might involve (Savage, 1987).

Referral

Given that most persistent changes in sexual interest and response tend to be multi-factorial in origin, patients with a persisting impairment of sexual function should, ideally, be referred to a sexual dysfunction clinic, where optimum assessment and treatment can be provided by a multi-disciplinary team (Gregoire, 1999a). The provision of such clinics within the British National Health Service (NHS), however, is patchy and most patients will be referred to services that have one particular approach. Gregoire (1999a) remarks that the choice of where to refer a patient will have a critical effect on both treatment approach and possible outcome. Before any appropriate course of action can be offered, the severity of the problem and its importance to the patient need to be ascertained (Ramage, 1998). Practitioners may find the following questions useful when thinking about what help might be most appropriate for a patient with a sexual dysfunction.

When and how did the problem start?

Sexual dysfunctions may be either primary or secondary. The term 'primary' is used to refer to sexual problems that have been present from the onset of sexual activity and the term 'secondary' to refer to problems that have developed after a period of satisfactory sexual activity. A sexual problem with a gradual onset, especially in the absence of any general relationship difficulties, points to an underlying physical cause (Watson and Davies, 1997).

Does the patient indicate that there were any potential precipitating factors?

As noted in Chapter 4, there are a number of 'life events' and other psychosocial factors that may act as possible precipitants for sexual problems. It is important to be particularly alert for those that involve loss or threaten a patient's self-image or the stability of his or her primary relationships. If such factors are reported and there are no indicators of ill-health, a more psychotherapeutic approach may be indicated.

In what situations does the problem occur?

Sexual dysfunctions may be either 'total' (sometimes also referred to as 'global'), or 'situational'. A sexual difficulty that is 'total' is one that occurs in all situations, whereas a 'situational' sexual problem is one that occurs in certain situations (e.g. penetrative sex with a partner) but not in others (e.g. when masturbating). Sexual problems that are situational tend to suggest a predominantly psychological or psychosocial cause.

Are there any indications of relationship difficulties?

Watson and Davies (1997) suggest that most relationship problems include difficulties with communication, conflict or commitment. However, Watson and Davies (1997) also state that while it is often easy to specify sexual aspects of a problem, relationship difficulties may be difficult to evaluate in a brief assessment. The 'relational' nature of certain sexual problems, such as differences in sexual interest, indicates the need for a treatment approach that will involve some reference to the couple and their relationship (Daines and Perrett, 2000). Where general relationship difficulties are indicated by a patient, referral of both the patient and his or her partner for couple or relationship counselling may be helpful (Catalan et al., 1990).

Are their any indicators of an underlying medical problem?

Ideally, all patients presenting with a persisting problem of sexual function should visit their GP for medical assessment and investigation, although some patients may be very reluctant to do so (Dean, 1998). As noted above, a sexual dysfunction of gradual onset in the absence of relationship difficulties often indicates a physical cause and as discussed in Chapter 4, there are a number of medical conditions and medications that may adversely affect sexual functioning. Bancroft (1989, p. 417 and p. 424) considers that the following should be considered indicators for the medical examination and investigation.

Female patients:

- Pain or discomfort during sexual activity.
- Recent onset of loss of sexual interest with no apparent cause.
- Recent history of ill-health or physical symptoms apart from the sexual problem.
- History of irregular menstruation or fertility problems.
- History of endocrine disorder or abnormal puberty.
- Peri- or post-menopausal women who are experiencing a sexual problem.
- The patient believes that a physical cause is likely or thinks that there is something abnormal with her genitalia.

Male patients:

- Pain or discomfort associated with sexual activity.
- Recent onset of loss of sexual interest with no apparent cause.
- Recent history of ill-health or physical symptoms apart from the sexual problem.
- History of endocrine disorder, genital problems (e.g. orchitis, torsion of the testes) or abnormal puberty.
- The patient believes a physical cause is likely or expresses concerns about his body or genitalia.
- Any man aged over 50 who is experiencing a sexual problem.

Bancroft (1989) also notes that the recognition of depression is particularly important. Depression may cause loss of interest in sex or may be a consequence of relationship or sexual difficulties. Where depression is severe, referral to a mental health care team may be indicated.

Biomedical interventions in the management of sexual dysfunction

Increasingly, through technological and pharmacological advances, medicine is assuming a greater role in the treatment of sexual dysfunctions (Tiefer, 1994; Hart and Wellings, 2002). Medical strategies to improve sexual functioning include the following.

Correction of iatrogenic sexual dysfunction

Where it is likely that prescribed medication is a causative factor in a sexual dysfunction, physicians may recommend that patients:

- Discontinue the drug.
- Reduce the dose.
- Postpone the daily dose until after sexual activity.
- Substitute an alternative drug.
- Use adjunctive agents to try to reduce side-effects (Wylie, 1998; Gregoire, 1999a).

Treatment of underlying medical conditions

The effective medical management of a number of underlying medical conditions may indirectly ameliorate sexual dysfunction (*see* Chapter 4). Certain sexual dysfunctions are more commonly caused by physical factors, for example, the majority of cases of dyspareunia in women are due to identifiable organic causes (e.g. endometriosis, vulval dysplasia, post-episiotomy scar tissue, vaginal infections) and will require appropriate gynaecological management. Wylie (1998) suggests that discomfort associated with penile penetration affects one in seven women over 35 years old and is usually the result of vaginal dryness. He notes that failure to treat this appropriately can lead to loss of sexual interest.

Treatments for specific sexual dysfunctions

The sexual dysfunction that has received most medical attention is erectile dysfunction. Recent UK guidelines detail the recommendations for the assessment, examination, and investigation of men presenting with erectile problems (Ralph and McNicholas, 2000) and recommend that any health professional discussing treatment options with a patient should ensure that:

- Unbiased information is offered on all available treatments, including the merits and known significant risks associated with each treatment option.
- The final choice of treatment is tailored to meet the needs of the patient.
- Agreed treatment goals are established from the commencement of treatment.

The treatment options listed in the guidelines include:

- Psychosexual therapy.
- Oral sildenafil (Viagra).
- Intra-cavernosal prostaglandin (alprostadil) injections.
- Trans-urethral alprostadil (MUSE).
- Vacuum devices.
- Penile prostheses.

The advantages and disadvantages of each of the above methods are also outlined by Ralph and McNicholas (2000) and recognition is given to the role of specialist nurses in both informing patients, and in initiating and monitoring therapy.

Medical interventions feature less prominently in the management of other sexual dysfunctions, although again there is a general bias towards male sexual problems. Topical anaesthetic sprays and gels and oral clomipramine have been used for several decades as treatments for premature ejaculation. The use of serotonin re-uptake inhibitors, such as paroxetine and fluoxetine, may also benefit some patients with premature ejaculation (Wylie, 1998). Interventions to ameliorate arousal and orgasmic difficulties in women have tended to be less pharmacologically orientated. They include Kegel exercises to strengthen the pubococcygeus muscle (to improve sensation and response) or a variation on this using vaginal cones (developed for stress incontinence) to increase pelvic muscle tone and awareness of sensations of the lower vagina and vulva (Wylie, 1998). Segraves and Segraves (1998) note that there is minimal evidence regarding pharmacotherapy for female sexual dysfunction. However, recent research concerning the use of sildenafil in pre-menopausal women with sexual arousal difficulties indicates that sildenafil may not only improve sexual arousal but also – indirectly – other aspects of a woman's sexual life (Caruso et al., 2001).

There are, however, limitations in the use of medical treatments for sexual dysfunction. Such interventions are only likely to help if they are acceptable to the patients and their sexual partners and are relatively free of undesirable side-effects. The difficulties associated with vacuum erection devices and intra-cavernosal injections mean that, to some men and their partners, these methods may be unacceptable. Priapism, one of the potential side-effects of intra-cavernosal injections may worsen a patient's erectile function if it is not rectified swiftly. Up to 10% of patients with penile prostheses may experience complications, including pain, mechanical failure and sepsis (Wylie, 1998). Although the use of oral treatments, such as sildenafil and apomorphine hydrochloride (used sub-lingually), are often more acceptable to patients they may cause unpleasant side-effects and their use is contraindicated for certain patients.

Attention to the psychological and interpersonal aspects of a patient's sexual problem remains an important aspect of the medical management of psychosexual problems. Medical treatments that restore sexual function do not necessarily restore sexual interest. Neither are such interventions a panacea for interpersonal difficulties, and a medical 'quick fix' will not necessarily promote or ensure intimacy in a relationship (Southern, 1999; Hart and Wellings, 2002). Segraves and Segraves (1998) observe that individuals who are experiencing relationship difficulties will often attempt to minimize these and point to a sexual complaint as the primary problem. Consequently, unacknowledged interpersonal difficulties may negate any beneficial effects afforded by treatment and some patients may actually stop such treatment when they realize that restoration of sexual function is not the solution to their problems. Furthermore, for some couples the restoration of physiological sexual functioning may actually create new tensions by disturbing the psychological equilibrium within the relationship (Daines and Perrett, 2000). Thus, it is not uncommon for psychosexual therapy to be offered in conjunction with any medical treatment.

Psychosexual therapy

The term 'psychosexual therapy' can denote one of a number of different psychological approaches to helping patients with sexual dysfunctions, including behaviour therapy (Masters and Johnson, 1976), cognitive behavioural therapy (Spence, 1991), behavioural-systems approaches (Crowe and Ridley, 2000), rational emotive therapy (Ellis and Dryden, 1999) and psychodynamic approaches (Daines and Perrett, 2000). In practice, however, much psychosexual therapy is characterized by a degree of eclecticism (Cooper, 1988). Probably the two most common types of psychosexual therapy provided within the British NHS are sex therapy and psychosexual medicine.

Sex therapy

The origins of modern sex therapy lie in the work of Masters and Johnson (1966, 1970) and Kaplan (1974, 1979). Cooper (1988) describes the approach of Masters and Johnson (1966, 1970) as partly behavioural in its origin and concepts, partly educational and partly 'permission-giving'. One of the central premises of this approach is that fear, in the form of performance anxiety, and failure to communicate are major factors in many sexual dysfunctions that are predominantly psychogenic in origin. To address this these authors developed the 'sensate focus' technique. This technique consists of a series of 'homework' exercises designed to help couples become more comfortable with physical contact and closeness. Its first phase involves exercises with a 'non-genital' genital focus. This is then followed by 'genital' sensate focus exercises in which touching and stimulating the genitals is permissible, but sexual intercourse is still prohibited. The work of Kaplan (1974) extends some of the ideas of Masters and Johnson (1966, 1970) by distinguishing between 'immediate' and 'remote' causes of sexual dysfunction. Kaplan's (1974, 1979) approach to psychosexual therapy aims not only to help people by using behavioural methods to recognize the 'here and now' patterns and causes of their sexual difficulties but also to develop deeper developmental insights where necessary. The latter is achieved by working with 'resistances' or 'defences' in both the individual and the couple as these emerge as blocks to the behavioural aspects of treatment.

Sex therapy predominantly involves working with couples, although some of its principles may be adapted and applied to working with individuals (*see* Hawton, 1985). Sex therapy begins with a careful assessment of the couple to determine their suitability for treatment. According to Hawton (1995, p. 308) factors that indicate a couple's suitability for sex therapy include:

- The sexual problem has continued for at least a few months.
- The likelihood that the problem is caused or is being maintained by psychological factors (even though physical factors may also be contributing to the problem).
- The sexual problem is not secondary to any general relationship difficulties.
- Sufficient harmony exists in the couple's general relationship to enable them to work collaboratively.
- Neither partner has a current major psychiatric illness.
- There is no serious alcohol or drug abuse.
- Female partners are not pregnant.
- Each partner shows reasonable motivation for treatment.

After assessing the couple's suitability for treatment, the therapist then presents a formulation of the problem, based on a detailed assessment, with a tentative outline of the possible maintaining factors. In 'standard' sex therapy, treatment is a combination of graded homework assignments, counselling (when 'blocks' arise in the homework assignments) and education (*see* Hawton, 1985; Bancroft, 1989; Spence, 1991). Treatment sessions usually occur weekly, at least at the onset of therapy, and the treatment programme normally lasts between eight and 20 sessions (Hawton, 1995).

Psychosexual medicine

Practitioners of psychosexual medicine are qualified doctors who have undertaken post-registration training with the Institute of Psychosexual Medicine (*see* Mathers et al., 1994). The focus of their work is on understanding how emotional factors, not always at a conscious level, interfere with sexual enjoyment and activity. A combination of specific listening skills, genital examination (when appropriate) and interpretation characterize this brief psychotherapeutic approach – sometimes also referred to as a 'psychosomatic approach' – which has its origins in the work of Michael Balint and Tom Main (Tunnadine, 1999). One of the assumptions of this approach is that the underlying causes of a sexual problem may be physical or psychological to varying proportions but are seldom limited only to one or the other. Aside from excluding physical pathology or abnormality, the genital examination is viewed as an important 'therapeutic' intervention in that patients' attitudes, anxieties and fantasies revealed at the time of this examination are often relevant to understanding their sexual problems. In addition to the psychosomatic genital examination, the other cornerstone of psychosexual medicine is the doctor–patient relationship (Botell, 2001). During each consultation, the practitioner of psychosexual medicine tries to give total attention to his or her patient's responses and behaviours while endeavouring to be aware of her or his own subjective reactions to the patient and to think about the meaning of what has taken place during the consultation. The aim of this approach is for the doctor to use information gained from the 'here and now' interaction of the doctor–patient relationship to enable patients themselves to discover the origins of their difficulties and solutions for their problems. Consequently, practitioners of psychosexual medicine usually work with individual patients rather than couples, although some practitioners may adapt their technique for work with couples on occasions (Gabbott et al., 1999; Pollen, 1999). According to the prospectus of the Institute of Psychosexual Medicine (IPM, 1995), the types of problem managed successfully by physicians skilled in this approach include:

- Non-consummation or dyspareunia.
- Erectile, ejaculatory and other penile problems, such as pain.

- Difficulties caused by the effects of illness, disability or ageing on sexuality.
- Lack of sexual interest, arousal or orgasm.
- Chronic pelvic pain, genital pain or recurrent discharge with or without a physical cause.
- Contraceptive-related problems.
- Difficulties associated with sexuality and terminal care.
- Sexual abuse.

The most important factor when deciding whether a patient is suitable for referral to a psychosexual medicine clinic is the extent to which he or she accepts that sex is a psychosomatic event, as the work will involve the examination of his or her feelings (Hutchinson, 2001). The patient also needs to understand that he or she will be doing the work both during and between consultations rather than waiting 'to be cured' by the doctor. Finally, practitioners of psychosexual medicine are trained to look specifically at the sexual area of a patient's life, most practitioners have little or no training in psychiatry or marital therapy. Hutchinson (2001) suggests that for patients to be helped by psychosexual medical practitioners, they need to be functioning reasonably 'normally' in other areas of their lives. She suggests that patients with personality disorders or a current psychiatric illness, couples with relationship difficulties, and individuals with gender identity problems are unlikely to benefit from psychosexual medicine.

The efficacy of psychosexual therapy

Rosen and Leiblum (1995) note that despite the conceptual and technical sophistication of current approaches to the treatment of sexual problems, the outcome of treatment is often less than satisfactory. These authors also observe that there is a paucity of methodologically robust research concerning the long-term outcomes of psychosexual therapy or the efficacy of psychological approaches compared to biomedical treatment. This seems to be supported by a recent review of interventions for vaginismus in which only two controlled trials were identified, although data were available from only one (McGuire and Hawton, 2001). However, Hawton (1995), in a review of the literature concerning sex therapy and other treatments for sexual dysfunction, suggests that:

> the format of effective conjoint sex therapy is now fairly clear and there is a good
> understanding of the sexual dysfunctions that respond best to this treatment and the
> couples most likely to benefit. (Hawton, 1995, p. 307)

In terms of the short-term effects of sex therapy, there appear to be marked differences in the response of different sexual dysfunctions to sex therapy. Hawton (1995, p. 308) observes that an 'excellent response' is obtained for vaginismus, and a 'good outcome in a substantial majority of cases of erectile dysfunction of psychogenic origin'. Treatment for impaired sexual desire, however, would appear to generate more variable initial outcome results and the outcome is often poor when this is a problem in men.

Crowe (1998) remarks that he rarely uses the word 'cure' when discussing sexual therapy, preferring to discuss the outcome of such treatment in terms of 'adjustment to' or 'coping with' sexual problems. He is of the opinion that there is only one area of sexual therapy where it is possible to refer to a cure with a minimal risk of relapse and that is in relation to couples who have been successful in their treatment for vaginismus.

Focus for intervention: the individual or the couple?

In sex therapy it is the couple that provides the focus of therapeutic endeavour, although sometimes during sex therapy with couples there may be issues, such as childhood sexual abuse, where it may be preferable to engage in work with an individual (Crowe, 1998). Hawton (1985) acknowledges that there are some sexual problems – primary orgasmic failure and primary ejaculatory failure – which may, at least initially, be more easily treated on an individual basis. There is, however, a general consensus that problems concerning levels of sexual interest can rarely be successfully addressed on an individual basis (Hawton, 1985; Crowe, 1998). A significant proportion of people seeking help for sexual dysfunctions do so without partners, either because they do not have a current partner or their current partner refuses to attend (Catalan et al., 1991). Sex therapy approaches have been developed for working with individuals, although the efficacy of many of these approaches has yet to be established (Hawton, 1985). Research by Stravynski et al. (1997), comparing the effects of two treatment approaches for 69 single men, suggests that treatment which pays attention to patients' interpersonal difficulties as well as their sexual dysfunction may result in better outcomes than approaches that concentrate on sexual functioning alone.

Psychosexual therapy or relationship counselling?

Psychosexual therapy will contain aspects of both sexual and relationship therapy (Gregory, 1999). For some practitioners, the treatment of sexual problems is just one aspect of relationship/couple therapy (Crowe and Ridley, 2000), whereas others view psychosexual therapy as being distinct from sexual and relationship counselling (Butler and Joyce, 1998). Hawton (1985) considers that couples whose sexual problems are the result of major difficulties in their general relationship are unlikely to be suitable for sex therapy. Indeed, Hawton (1995) suggests that the factors related to a good prognosis in sex therapy include:

- The quality of the couple's relationship.
- The motivation of the partners (in particular, male partners).
- Physical attraction between partners.

If couples seek help for a sexual dysfunction but their general relationship is very disturbed, it may be better if general relationship difficulties are addressed before proceeding with psychotherapeutic interventions for their sexual problems. On occasions, however, it can be quite difficult even for experienced psychosexual therapists and relationship counsellors to determine initially whether a couple's sexual problems are the consequence of general relationship difficulties or vice versa.

Providers of psychosexual therapy

Psychosexual therapy services will vary from one area to another, and a list of clinics and individual psychosexual therapists can be obtained from the British Association for Sexual and Relationship Therapy (*see* Appendix I). Within the NHS, a number of professional groups and agencies may provide sex therapy, including:

- Sexual dysfunction clinics.
- Clinical psychologists.
- Departments of psychiatry.
- Genitourinary medicine clinics.
- Family planning clinics.
- Specially trained practitioners working in a variety of different settings.

Sexual dysfunction clinics are few in number and waiting lists can be long. Gregoire (1999b) notes that many psychiatry departments now rarely do any work with sexual problems as priority tends to be given to serious mental illness. A number of genitourinary medicine clinics may offer psychosexual therapy services (Keane et al., 1997; Kell, 2001) and patients are able to refer themselves directly to such clinics. As with genitourinary medicine clinics, patients can usually refer themselves directly to family planning clinics and many of these clinics will have physicians trained in psychosexual medicine or referral pathways to psychosexual medicine clinics. Doctors trained in psychosexual medicine may also work in other areas, such as general practice, urology, genitourinary medicine and gynaecology – a full list of current providers of psychosexual medicine is available from the Institute of Psychosexual Medicine (*see* Appendix I).

Outside the NHS, the largest provider of psychosexual therapy is the charitable organization Relate (formerly known as the Marriage Guidance Council). In addition to providing psychosexual therapy at over a hundred locations within the UK (Cole, 1997), Relate is also the largest provider of relationship counselling services, and therefore may be particularly useful for patients where relationship difficulties may be contributing significantly to psychosexual problems and vice versa. Patients usually refer themselves directly to Relate but need to be aware that the focus of Relate's work tends to be with couples (both heterosexual and homosexual) and a fee is charged by the organization for its services.

Key points of Chapter 5

- Sexual dysfunction is a term that is used to describe the persistent impairment of normal patterns of sexual interest and response.
- Sexual dysfunctions are often classified according to the stage of sexual response that is affected.
- A sexual dysfunction may have always been present (primary), or may develop after a period of satisfactory sexual activity (secondary); some sexual problems occur every time sexual activity is attempted (total), whereas as others occur only in certain situations (situational).
- Current conventional classification systems of sexual dysfunction do not adequately reflect the variety and type of sexual problems encountered in clinical practice.
- Sexual function in conventional classification systems is often equated solely with penile–vaginal intercourse culminating in orgasm. The

dichotomous view of sexual health as being either functional or dysfunctional also neglects the importance of sexual satisfaction.

- Sexual dysfunctions usually occur as a consequence of a combination of organic, psychological, and interpersonal factors. The significance of each of these factors in the aetiology and maintenance of a sexual problem will vary between individuals and the effective management of such problems will need to reflect this.

- Patients with sexual dysfunctions require specialist assessment and treatment.

- Ideally, all patients presenting with a persisting impairment of sexual function (particularly if the problem is of a gradual onset and occurs in the absence of general relationship difficulties) should attend for medical assessment and investigation to exclude any underlying pathology.

- Although not providers of psychosexual therapy, it is important that practitioners are able to recognize when referral is appropriate and discuss with patients what such treatment might involve.

- Potential sources of specialist help for patients with sexual dysfunction include sexual dysfunction clinics, psychosexual medicine clinics, genitourinary and family planning clinics which provide psychosexual counselling and therapy services, and the charitable organization, Relate.

Key reading

Hawton, K. (1995) Treatment of sexual dysfunction by sex therapy and other approaches. *British Journal of Psychiatry* **167**, 307–314.

Hutchinson, H. (2001) The psychosexual medicine clinic. In: Skrine, R., Montford, H. (eds). *Psychosexual Medicine: An Introduction* (second edition). London: Arnold.

PART II

PSYCHOSEXUAL ISSUES IN SEXUAL HEALTH CARE

CHAPTER 6

Reproductive sexual health

Introduction

The psychosexual aspects of reproductive sexual health are very varied. Psychosexual problems may be the consequence of fertility problems, pregnancy and peri-natal loss. Conversely, underlying psychosexual difficulties sometimes contribute to fertility and contraceptive problems or find expression in complaints about contraceptive methods or unplanned pregnancy. As reproductive health is intimately connected to the sense of self for many people, it is unsurprising that practitioners working in fertility and family planning clinics and maternity care frequently encounter patients with psychosexual anxiety and distress. For practitioners working in more general settings, psychosexual distress associated with reproductive health issues may manifest itself at other times in patients' lives, such as the menopause, or during gynaecological procedures or other intimate aspects of care commonly undertaken in health care settings.

Fertility problems

Problems with fertility affect approximately one in seven couples in the UK and are associated with deep psychological and emotional distress for many individuals. The diagnosis of impaired fertility is often a 'life crisis', the response to which is in part determined by how individuals have dealt with previous challenges in their lives (Rutter, 2000b). According to Rutter (2000b) feelings associated with the experience of impaired fertility include:

- Uncertainty.
- Injustice.
- Sense of failure – low self-esteem, inadequacy.

99

- Feelings of insecurity and loss of control.
- Isolation.
- Damaged or distorted body image associated with low sperm counts or tubal damage.
- Hidden loss.

Silman (1995) suggests that the expressed desire to have a child may contain within it a complex set of other desires, including:

- Being a parent.
- Satisfying the expectations of others.
- Proving the male partner's masculinity or the female patient's femininity.
- Attaining companionship in later life.

Hence, the hidden losses associated with impaired fertility may be very varied. Rutter (2000b) observes that these feelings often go 'deep to the heart' and often feel unspeakable because patients fear no-one will understand. Although the experience of impaired fertility is often construed as a loss, it may also be perceived as a threat. Glover et al. (1998) suggest that men's experiences of, and responses to, sub-fertility differ fundamentally from those of their partners. The men affected by sub-fertility in their study reported higher levels of persistent anxiety, feeling 'less of a man' and blamed themselves for their sub-fertility. Anxiety seemed to persist regardless of whether a child was subsequently born. Glover and colleagues (1998) consider that this anxiety suggests men perceive sub-fertility more in terms of threat than loss:

> If subfertility is perceived as a threatening event the experience of achieving a
> pregnancy or having a child will not necessarily restore feelings of manliness,
> especially if the child is achieved through assisted conception. (Glover et al., 1998,
> p. 1406)

Bor and Scher (1995) suggest that the high premium placed on having children by society, can mean that a diagnosis of impaired fertility leads to secrecy, shame and depression. They note that for some couples the social shame of sub-fertility may result in them choosing not to disclose this information to relatives and close friends. Consequently, some couples will feel isolated and will lack the support of relatives and close friends whilst undergoing the stressful process of investigation and treatment for their fertility problems.

Read (1999) notes that sub-fertility and sexual problems may be connected in two ways:

- Psychosexual problems may be contributory factors in apparent sub-fertility.
- The diagnosis, investigation and management of impaired fertility may precipitate or exacerbate sexual problems.

The stress of sub-fertility and its treatment may be a cause of sexual difficulties for both partners. Pressure to 'perform', arousal difficulties associated with anxiety and distress, and restricting sexual contact to times when there is the greatest chance of conception may all cause difficulties. Read (1999) observes that:

> These stresses all conspire to alienate the couple from the recreational aspects of sexual expression and focus them, sometimes obsessively, on the procreative aspect of sexual intercourse only. (Read, 1999, p. 587)

Concerns about funding treatment for fertility problems, may also exacerbate a couple's stress, particularly as the success rate for any one cycle of treatment tends to be low (Rutter, 2000b). Wylie (1994) notes that in addition to the 'goal-orientated approach' of having sexual contact only during times of perceived greater fertility, the anxieties associated with failure to conceive can generate blame and guilt in each partner, thereby straining their relationship still further. Consequently, this can lead to the avoidance of sexual activity even if a specific sexual dysfunction is not present. Importantly, recent guidelines recommend that couples should be advised to have regular intercourse throughout the menstrual cycle and not just at times when fertility is perceived to be greater (RCOG, 1999). Impaired fertility may also be the result of existing sexual difficulties, dysfunctions or preferences. Retrograde ejaculation and the absence of penile–vaginal penetrative intercourse are often associated with apparent sub-fertility (Read, 1999). Read (1999) observes that clear questions about a couple's sex life and sexual functioning, both before and after the diagnosis of impaired fertility, could spare them months or even years of invasive and expensive treatment.

Pregnancy

Pregnancy, childbirth and the transition to parenthood represent a fundamental period of change for prospective parents and the relationship that exists between them. Aston (2001) notes that a pregnant woman experiences a sudden alteration in her physiology, her body and her appearance, as well as her social status. Aston (2001) suggests that a degree of personal stress is a common feature of most pregnancies, and that pregnancy is sometimes accompanied by the revival of old conflicts and worries, as well as memories of childhood experiences of the relationship with one's own parents. Pregnancy can both disrupt and strengthen a couple's relationship, and sexual interaction is often one aspect of the relationship that is altered. The findings of recent study by Bartellas et al. (2000), suggest that vaginal intercourse and overall sexual activity decreases throughout pregnancy and that many women (58% of the women in the study by Bartellas et al., 2000) also report a decrease in sexual desire. There are likely to be a number of reasons for this. Sexual health is intimately linked to self-image, and changes in body shape and image occur rapidly in pregnancy. Some women (and their partners) view these changes very positively, whereas others do not, especially during the last three months of pregnancy (Aston, 2001). Aston (2001) also notes that tiredness, changes that occur to the breasts, backache and frequency of micturition are all physical changes that can adversely affect sexual interest and activity.

Anxieties about the possible adverse effects of sexual intercourse on pregnancy may also inhibit sexual activity. Bartellas et al. (2000) report that 49% of women in their study were worried that sexual intercourse may harm their pregnancy, expressing concerns that sexual activity might lead to pre-term delivery or premature rupture of the membranes. These concerns appear to increase as pregnancy progresses. Although there are indications for abstaining from sexual intercourse during pregnancy (Table 6.1), generally, there appears to be no significant increase in fetal problems in women who are sexually active throughout pregnancy (Read, 1999). However, some women do experience painful uterine contractions following orgasm. Once women have experienced this they tend to have sex less frequently or abstain completely (Savage and Reader, 1984).

Dyspareunia also appears to be a significant problem for some pregnant women and its prevalence appears to increase as pregnancy progresses. A number of psychological, interpersonal and physical factors (see Table 6.2 for examples of the latter) may alone, or in combination, lead to dyspareunia in pregnancy (Aston, 2001). Consequently, reports of sexual symptoms such as dyspareunia and the avoidance of sexual intercourse in pregnancy require careful evaluation by health care professionals (Aston, 2001).

Table 6.1: Indications for abstaining from sexual intercourse during pregnancy

Vaginal bleeding
Placenta praevia
Rupture of the membranes
Premature dilatation of the cervix
Engaged fetal head
Multiple pregnancy
History of premature delivery

(From Read, 1999; Aston, 2001.)

Table 6.2: Possible physical causes of dyspareunia

Pelvic and genital vasocongestion
Reduced vaginal lubrication
Subluxation of symphysis pubis and sacroiliac joints
Retroverted uterus
Chorioamnionitis
Candidal, trichomonal, herpetic and genital wart infections
Weight of partner on gravid uterus (in late pregnancy)
Deep engagement of fetal head

(From Aston, 2001)

Much of the research examining the possible impact of pregnancy on sexuality and sexual expression focuses on penile–vaginal sexual intercourse to the neglect of other forms of sexual intimacy, although work by Barclay et al. (1994) is an informative exception. Indeed, in much of the research on this subject sexual desire or interest is often equated solely with the willingness or otherwise of women to engage in penetrative vaginal intercourse (Hobbs et al., 1999). This neither reflects adequately the different forms of sexual expression of many heterosexual women nor recognizes that not all pregnant women are heterosexual, although this is often assumed to be so. Such an assumption in clinical practice can not only have a negative effect on a pregnant woman's sexual identity but also marginalize her partner's contribution to her ante-natal care (Aston, 2001).

In general, little attention in research has been given to the partners of pregnant women. Barclay et al. (1994) indicate that the substantial decline in sexual interest noted in many pregnant women is not always matched by that of their male partners. Such a mismatch of sexual interest could present a challenge to some couples, but studies of sexual interest and expression during pregnancy, however, rarely take into account the relationship context. Hobbs et al. (1999) note that although sexual activity or the lack of it can affect a couple's relationship there may also be other emotional changes during pregnancy which affect the sexual interest or satisfaction of either partner. The assumption that 'normal' couples enjoy regular and frequent sexual activity is just an assumption (Hobbs et al., 1999), and lack of sexual interest or infrequent sexual activity during pregnancy should not automatically be interpreted as a sign of sexual 'pathology' or a harbinger of relationship difficulties.

Rutter (2000a) considers that the management of labour and childbirth can profoundly affect a woman's subsequent feelings about sex. She suggests that the feelings a woman may have about her body after childbirth may be affected by the way she was treated during delivery, and suggests that anxieties about resuming sex can sometimes be the consequence of not being respected or feeling invaded at the time of delivery. Childbirth, for some women, may also evoke distressing memories of previous sexual assault and abuse (Kitzinger, 1992) or of previous traumatic experiences incurred as a result of undergoing invasive obstetric or gynaecological interventions (RCOG, 1997). Rutter (2000a) suggests that a traumatic delivery may generate fears about damage to the vagina and anxiety about resuming sex. Similarly, witnessing a traumatic birth can generate fears about causing pain or putting partners through the distress of childbirth again, which sometimes leads to psychosexual difficulties for men (O'Driscoll, 1994; Read, 1999; Rutter, 2000a).

Post-natal sexual problems seem to be a frequent occurrence. Over 80% of women in a study by Barrett et al. (2000) reported experiencing at least one sexual problem in the first three months after giving birth and two-thirds were still experiencing problems at six months after childbirth. The most frequetly cited problems were vaginal dryness, loss of sexual interest and dyspareunia. Dixon et al. (2000) report that 50% of the first-time parents in their study described their sex lives as 'poor' or 'not very good' eight months after the birth of their baby and one in five indicated they would like help for this. Sexual interest and responsiveness after childbirth cannot be isolated from the emotional, psychosocial and interpersonal adjustments that the transition to parenthood requires (*see* Raphael-Leff, 1991; Rutter, 2000a). Although some sexual symptoms may be the consequence of hormonal changes after childbirth which result in lower oestrogen and raised prolactin levels, the effects of fatigue associated with coping with a new baby, and anxieties about sex causing damage, should not be under-estimated.

Loss in pregnancy

Pregnancy, like most changes in life, involves both gain and loss. Being pregnant and becoming a parent inevitably means giving up certain aspects of one's identity or lifestyle. For some prospective parents, pregnancy is associated with a loss of freedom and independence. Some women may incur loss of income and on occasions, job, career and status as a consequence of becoming pregnant. For some women, pregnancy will generate fears about losing their sexual attractiveness and also constitutes a loss of privacy in that it is a very public manifestation of their sex life. There are other, often extremely traumatic, losses associated with pregnancy, such as ectopic pregnancy, miscarriage, termination of pregnancy, a child that is stillborn and neonatal death, that evoke considerable and sometimes long-lasting grief in those who are affected (Brien and Fairburn, 1996; Berry, 1999). Although traumatic, these losses may sometimes not be disclosed to others, leaving the individual or couple with a 'hidden loss' and often unresolved grief. This grief may sometimes emerge at a later date in the form of distress at the time of other 'life events'.

As already noted in chapters 1 and 4, loss changes the way individuals view themselves, including the sexual aspects of their self-concepts. Loss associated with reproduction, is likely to affect not only an individual's self-perception but also the perception a woman and her partner have of themselves as a couple. Peri-natal death is an area where grief and sex are intimately entwined and, consequently, psychosexual anxieties and relationship difficulties may accompany bereavement. Miscarriage, even in the very early weeks of pregnancy, is felt by many as a great loss and bereavement (Steele and Andrews, 2001) and although a relatively common outcome of pregnancy, can leave a couple feeling isolated both from those around them and from each other within their relationship. Raphael-Leff (1991) notes that:

> Communication may be impaired as each partner deals alone with complex feelings. Unconscious blame may fester in their relationship alongside unanswered questions about whose "fault" it is, whether miscarriage was triggered by sexual intercourse or she may be responsible for having broken some antenatal taboo, whether it occurred because of a previous abortion or is a "blighted pregnancy" which comes from his or her "side of the family". (Raphael-Leff, 1991, p. 439)

Raphael-Leff (1991) states that when a baby dies before the mother has had the opportunity to establish the baby as being separate from herself, the loss may be felt as a loss of part of her own physical being and potential. She notes that this 'vague undefined sense of dispossession and emptiness' can make grieving particularly difficult and that parents sometimes need help to define what is being mourned. Raphael-Leff (1991) also observes that pleasure in sex after a stillbirth can be inhibited by guilt and the association of sex with tragedy. She suggests that a 'vicious circle of defensive activity' to prevent mourning can be established as:

> Both sexual withdrawal for fear of another pregnancy and further loss and a compulsion to conceive in order to replace the dead baby prevent the couple drawing closer and sharing their grief during love-making. (Raphael-Leff, 1991, p. 640)

Termination of pregnancy for fetal abnormalities may evoke the same feelings as other forms of peri-natal death but is often complicated by the fact that the termination of pregnancy is chosen. One or both parents may feel guilt not only at having made this decision but also because they were not prepared to look after a disabled child. Brien and Fairbairn (1996) note that for couples in this situation:

> In truth there are two deaths that are grieved; first the death of hopes for the perfect baby that occur when the results were given, and later the actual death of the abnormal baby. The couple also suffer the loss of their own sense of themselves. (Brien and Fairbairn, 1996, p. 134)

Although sex may become connected with the pain and distress of reproduction, Brien and Fairbairn (1996) point out that within a couple there may be differences in each partner's attitudes to sex. Whereas one partner may associate sex with traumatic pregnancy and therefore view it as something to be feared, the other may find it a source of comfort and closeness. It is not difficult to see how at such periods of extreme stress, sexual difficulties may quickly develop into relationship problems.

Although not all unplanned pregnancies are unwanted pregnancies, for some women an unplanned pregnancy may be an unwelcome event in her life. On other occasions, a planned pregnancy may, because of a change in personal circumstances, become unwanted. In both of these situations a woman may request a termination of her pregnancy. Although only a small minority of women would appear to experience long-term adverse psychological sequelae after an abortion (Zolese and Blacker, 1992), for some women there may be feelings of loss, guilt, sadness or emptiness (Rutter, 2000a). Any expression of sadness or grief may be blocked for some women by the perception that they do not have the right to mourn, or the fear that any expression of such feelings will be interpreted as them having made the wrong decision (Brien and Fairburn, 1996). Sexual problems can develop after an abortion for a variety of different reasons. These include the continual association of sexual activity with abortion, the fear that an unwanted pregnancy could happen again (particularly if there has been a contraceptive failure) and unspoken anger and hurt between a couple that finds expression in the form of sexual dysfunction (Brien and Fairbairn, 1996).

Contraception

Decisions about contraception are often multifaceted. In addition to choosing which method and who should use it, contraceptive choice also involves decisions about whether or not to have children and if children are desired, decisions about the timing of their birth and how many children to have. Roberts (1993) observes that:

> Patients bring to even the most apparently uncomplicated consultation their own hidden agenda, which doctors and nurses, intent on the rational and scientific aspects of birth control, frequently miss. (Roberts, 1993, p. 21)

Unsurprisingly, decisions about the control of fertility and reproduction may become both a source and a manifestation of conflict. Christopher (1993) notes that conflicts may manifest themselves in a number of different ways, including:

- Complaints or expressed dissatisfaction with all contraceptive methods.
- Complaints about a method that has previously been acceptable and used seemingly without problem.
- Erratic use of a contraceptive method (especially in a patient who has previously managed to use a method satisfactorily).
- Shifting from a more 'reliable' method of contraception to a less effective one.

Christopher (1993) states that when faced with a patient who expresses dissatisfaction with all available methods of contraception, it is important that practitioners give the patient space to talk rather than compelling her (or him) to make a choice. Christopher (1993) suggests that it may be necessary to challenge the patient directly with a statement that reflects the patient's apparent dissatisfaction with all methods, acknowledges the lack of an ideal method, and includes a tentative enquiry as to whether there is anything else troubling the patient. Christopher (1993) also suggests that erratic use of a contraceptive method and complaints about a previously satisfactory method of contraception should (once medical reasons for the problems have been excluded) warrant further exploration in order to identify and understand any conflicts that may be present. Sometimes such conflicts may not be in a patient's immediate personal awareness, for example, the shift from a more reliable method to a less effective one may reveal a covert desire to become pregnant, although this may be denied by the patient if asked (Christopher, 1993). The quality of a relationship and its stability is also likely to have a strong influence on contraceptive use (Christopher, 1993; Brien and Fairburn, 1996). Contraception is generally less likely to be used, or more likely to be used erratically, when there are changes going on, or instability in a relationship. Thus, the beginning and end of a relationship are times when the use of contraception may often be sporadic. Brien and Fairburn (1996) suggest that the 'sporadic' use of contraception is also more likely to occur in relationships when both partners are fighting for control. The use or non-use of contraception can be a way of trying to limit a partner's sexual activity or enjoyment of sex. Pregnancy following erratic contraceptive use can be used as a means of 'testing' a relationship or retaining a 'hold' over a partner. Pregnancy is often used to control women. Men who fear not being in control in a relationship, or who need to compensate for their own inadequacies, may seek to keep their partners pregnant and therefore dependent upon them (Christopher, 1993; Brien and Fairburn, 1996).

Consultations about contraception also provide opportunities for the disclosure of overt or covert sexual problems (Wakley, 1993). On occasions, a contraceptive method will be blamed for sexual symptoms that have their true origins in feelings that cannot be expressed openly. Although hormonal methods of contraception may alter mood and sexual interest in some, Christopher (1993) considers that such alterations may be related to other issues, for example:

- The contraceptive method is too effective, thereby removing an element of risk from sexual activity that some people enjoy.
- Difficulties associated with refusing the sexual advances of partners.
- Interpersonal difficulties in the relationship such as anger or resentment.

Although possible medical reasons for symptoms need to be excluded, blaming the contraceptive method can be a way for some patients to redefine interpersonal difficulties as a 'medical problem', and one for the health professional to solve. Roberts (1993) notes that every contraceptive method has a different meaning for each individual patient and the same is true for unplanned pregnancy. Although every patient is unique, it is sometimes possible to recognize patterns of unspoken messages that are conveyed by pregnancy. Brien and Fairbairn (1996, pp 14–15) write that, 'pregnancy can be a sign of distress and may also have a purpose, it can often be an imaginary solution to complex personal problems'. For some women, a baby may be perceived as the answer to being unloved and uncared for. For others, having a baby establishes their fertility, femininity and identity. Christopher (1993) remarks that men who feel socially inadequate may put great emphasis on their ability to get their partner pregnant. Pregnancy may also happen when a woman is faced with a difficult or painful choice, providing her with a means of avoiding the responsibility for making a decision, or offering a possible solution to conflicts with a partner or family (Brien and Fairbairn, 1996). For some, however, once the pregnancy is confirmed and the reality of coping with a baby is faced, abortion is requested. Thus a request for an abortion can sometimes be a symptom of underlying distress or conflict.

Repeat abortions account for 10% of all abortions, and although no contraceptive method is perfect, repeated unwanted pregnancy may sometimes be a symptom of deeper difficulties or anxieties. Christopher (1993) observes that shame and guilt related to past sexual relationships and behaviours are important emotions in contraceptive practice. Consequently, a previous unplanned pregnancy and abortion will not always lead to more careful contraceptive use 'as there may be an unconscious wish to deny what has happened and to get pregnant again to make some kind of reparation' (Christopher, 1993, p. 11). Although a woman's unconscious wish may be for further pregnancy to resolve the feelings of loss or guilt associated with a previous abortion, often external constraints and pressures have not changed. According to Brien and Fairbairn (1996), this may consequently lead to either a pregnancy or baby that is not wanted in its own right, or another abortion which merely compounds a woman's sense of loss still further. Sometimes the experience of undergoing an abortion generates fears about impaired fertility and getting pregnant again may for some women be a way of trying to dispel such anxieties. Unfortunately, however, a further pregnancy that ends in abortion will only cause these anxieties to grow unless they are recognized and explored (Brien and Fairburn, 1996). Brien and Fairbairn (1996) suggest that esteem, or the lack of it, is often a predisposing factor for multiple unwanted pregnancies. These authors contend that when a woman feels worthless she cares little about what happens to her and that this may manifest itself in her attitude to her own sexual health. The request for another abortion and the concomitant unsympathetic responses that can be evoked in health professionals by a woman's seemingly uncaring attitude merely reinforces this sense of personal worthlessness. Women requesting an abortion, particularly repeat abortions may generate very difficult feelings in practitioners that make it difficult to stay alongside the patient and retain psychosexual awareness. However, it is important to note that for some women the request for an abortion may provide 'the only window to her feelings about herself, particularly when these are protected by layers of aggression' (Brien and Fairbairn, 1996, p. 121).

Key points of Chapter 6

- Psychosexual problems may contribute to sub-fertility and may also be sequelae of the investigation and treatment of fertility problems.
- The changes associated with pregnancy, childbirth and the transition to parenthood may alter the way in which individuals view themselves and how a couple views their relationship.
- Although there are indications for abstaining from sexual intercourse during pregnancy, for most pregnant women sexual intercourse throughout pregnancy is possible. However, many women and their partners worry that sexual activity may affect pregnancy adversely and will benefit from being able to discuss these anxieties with health professionals.
- Sexual interest appears to decline for some women as pregnancy progresses, although this is not necessarily the case for their partners.
- Reports of sexual symptoms, such as dyspareunia and the avoidance of sexual activity during pregnancy, require careful and systematic evaluation by practitioners.
- A large proportion of women report sexual problems post-natally. Vaginal dryness, loss of sexual interest and dyspareunia are common problems.
- Childbirth may evoke distressing memories for some women of previous traumatic experiences. The feelings a woman may have about her body and the sexual aspects of her self-image after childbirth may also be altered by adverse experiences during childbirth.
- Ectopic pregnancy, miscarriage, termination of pregnancy, stillbirth and neonatal death may all lead to an alteration in sexual interest and response if sex becomes associated with tragedy, guilt or fear.

- Complaints about and difficulties associated with the use of contraception may sometimes serve as indicators of underlying conflict, anxiety or distress, as may an unplanned pregnancy.

Key reading

Aston, G. (2001) Sexuality during pregnancy. In: Andrews, G. (ed.). *Women's Sexual Health* (second edition). London: Baillière Tindall.

Christopher, E. (1993) Unconscious factors in contraceptive care: understanding ambivalence and poor motivation. In: Montford, H., Skrine, R. (eds). *Contraceptive Care: Meeting Individual Needs*. London: Chapman & Hall.

CHAPTER 7

Sexual orientation

Introduction

Sexual orientation cannot simply be equated with sexual behaviour. A person will have a sexual or erotic orientation irrespective of whether he or she has ever had sexual contact with another individual. Some people who identify as heterosexual on occasions feel attracted to or have sexual relationships with persons of the same gender, just as some people who identify as gay or lesbian on occasions feel attracted to or have sexual relationships with persons of the opposite gender. There is a tendency in society towards a bipolar categorization of sexuality, where the possibility of being attracted to both genders either simultaneously or sequentially is not generally acknowledged; consequently, the labels used to describe sexual orientation do not always reflect an individual's erotic orientation adequately. As Hitchings (1997, p. 303) writes, 'the terms lesbian, gay, bisexual and heterosexual are best considered as abstractions. Each person has a unique sexuality that is lost in categorization'.

Being gay, lesbian or bisexual is not a sexual problem. Psychosexual difficulties for some people may arise, however, around creating and sustaining a sexual identity that values homoerotic desire, and maintaining sexually satisfying and loving relationships in a society, where homophobia and heterosexism prevail.

Same-sex desire

Given that 'dominant societal discourses make no secret of the fact that homosexuality is a minority concern to be tolerated but not accepted' (Tasker and McCann, 1999, p. 33), it is perhaps not surprising that anxiety often accompanies the awareness of homoerotic desire. All those individuals who do eventually identify as gay, lesbian or bisexual will at some level have absorbed the cultural expectation of heterosexuality. They will have grown up in a society which prizes heterosexuality over homosexuality and bisexuality, and actively promotes stereotyped, negative and misleading images of gay men and lesbians (Gordon, 1988; Davies, 1996a).

Many gay and lesbian adults report having had an early sense of being different from their peers (*see* Tasker and McCann, 1999). Subsequent awareness of homoerotic desire may provide some individuals with an explanation for such feelings and consequently a gay, lesbian or bisexual identity will be both accepted and welcomed. For others, same-gender attraction will lead to denial or avoidance of a non-heterosexual identity. Examples of this may include exaggerated 'gender typical' behaviours, the verbal and physical abuse of others who are perceived to be gay or lesbian, a precipitous marriage or requesting professional help to 'change' their sexual orientation.

For some individuals, the conflict between an awareness of their own sexual orientation and the values of a society where heterosexism and homophobia prevail, creates almost unbearable anxiety and tension which eventually finds expression in a variety of emotional and behavioural problems. Such problems may include generalized anxiety, phobias, psychosomatic illnesses, depression, alcohol and substance misuse, and other forms of self-harm, including unsafe sex and attempted suicide. Anxieties relating to sexual orientation may present in a number of covert ways, including relationship and sexual difficulties. In such circumstances it is not the individual's sexual orientation that is the problem, but heterosexism and (actual or anticipated) homophobia that generate distress. For practitioners who encounter individuals who are uncertain of their sexual orientation, questions such as *'Am I gay?'* are impossible to answer. In such situations it is important to allow patients to explore their feelings and thoughts about their sexuality without any prejudice on the part of the practitioner as to which orientation they should develop (Hitchings, 1997).

Coming out

For individuals who do identify as bisexual, lesbian or gay, there is likely to be considerable apprehension about whether to be open about their bisexual or homosexual orientation. Expression of homosexual orientation may incur opprobrium, rejection, discrimination and, on occasions, violence (*see* Mason and Palmer, 1996), whereas maintaining a public persona of heterosexuality may cause tension and a relentless fear of being 'found out'. The fragmentation of one's sexual identity between private and public spheres may in turn lead to a split between emotions and behaviour making it difficult for an individual to experience sexual and emotional intimacy concurrently.

'Coming out' is the term used to describe a life-long process which starts with 'coming out to oneself' and for many individuals involves informing others of their sexual orientation. The intrapsychic and interpersonal transformations that constitute this process are influenced by a number of factors including gender, race or ethnicity, the attitudes and values prevailing in society at the time, location (particularly the significance of urban versus rural residency), family background, physical disability and sensory impairment (Davies, 1996b).

It is not uncommon for lesbian and gay young people who 'come out' to their families to be rejected or mistreated by family members (Trenchard and Warren, 1984). Therefore, for young people who are contemplating 'coming out', issues such as personal safety (protection from abuse by family members), housing (if they are forced to leave the family home) and access to peer support need to be considered (Davies, 1996c). Counselling, in the form of family or systemic therapy, may be useful for some adolescents with issues relating to their sexual identity (*see* Tasker and McCann, 1999). A sizable minority of people, however, will not become aware of their homoerotic orientation until later in life, when they are married and/or parents. Bell (1999) remarks that such people often require 'careful and compassionate counselling'.

Hitchings (1997) observes that it is particularly important that people who are beginning the process of 'coming out' to others, choose to tell first people who are most likely to be validating of their sexuality. Making people aware of their local lesbian and gay switchboard and support organizations may help to ensure this. Hitchings (1997) also suggests that it is useful to remind people who are 'coming out' that although negative responses from family members can be particularly painful, the reactions of family and friends can move in a more positive direction given time.

Whether 'coming out' or not has a direct effect on an individual's health is still uncertain (*see* Cole et al. 1996; Taylor, 1999). Non-disclosure of one's sexual orientation, however, may indirectly affect one's sexual and general health when it restricts access to appropriate care, advice and support (Taylor, 1999; Platzer and James, 2000). There are a number of reasons why patients who are bisexual, lesbian or gay choose not to share this information with health professionals, including:

- The presumption of heterosexuality that many health professionals convey in their initial encounters with patients.
- Previous experience of voyeuristic and abusive reactions from health professions following such disclosure.
- Anticipation of hostility, rejection or embarrassment.

The reticence of some patients to disclose their sexual orientation may have little to do with their perception of health workers' attitudes or previous experience of health care, but may reflect concerns relating to the effect of such information on future applications for life insurance (Bell, 1999). Whatever the reasons, concerns about disclosing their sexual orientation will make it difficult for many gay men, lesbians and bisexuals to access appropriate help, advice and support for sexual anxieties or distress. Sadly, some patients who do trust health professionals with information about their sexual orientation find that it is their sexual orientation that becomes the focus of the practitioner's attention, and not the problems with which they present. Platzer and James (2000) report how one respondent in their study described:

> feeling humiliated and embarrassed when a practitioner conveyed negative and judgemental attitudes about her sexual identity during a consultation by suggesting that she had a problem and needed to see a psychosexual counsellor. The symptoms this woman described were those of an acute anxiety state, and the stress associated with the encounter disrupted her life for several weeks, putting a considerable strain on her relationship and her ability to function in her job. (Platzer and James, 2000, p. 197)

The pathologization of same-sex desire

There is no scientific basis for viewing homosexuality as a disease or lesbian, gay or bisexual individuals as being psychiatrically disturbed on the basis of their sexual orientation (Gonsiorek, 1982, McColl, 1994). Although homosexuality was declassified as a mental illness by the American Psychiatric Association as long ago as 1973, the experience of many gay men and lesbians, particularly with regard to mental health services, suggests that the pathological model of same-sex desire remains pervasive (Golding, 1997; MacFarlane, 1998; Bartlett et al., 2001). In the area of psychotherapy, the 'pathologizing' of gay men and lesbians seems especially prevalent among psychodynamic psychotherapists (Denman, 1993), although it also persists in a number of other therapeutic traditions (*see* Shelley, 1998; Milton and Coyle, 1999).

Although the 'disease model' of homosexuality has lost all scientific credibility, it still constitutes the basis of many of the 'conversion' or 'reparative/reorientation therapies' advocated by evangelical 'ex-gay' organizations and some adherents to certain schools of psychotherapy. There are no methodologically sound empirical data to support the claims made by proponents of 'conversion' and 'reorientation therapies' (*see* Haldemann, 1991; Schreier, 1998). Some commentators suggest that these approaches not only reflect and encourage societal prejudice against gay, lesbian and bisexual people, but actually may harm already vulnerable individuals (Haldemann, 1991; Hancock, 1995; Schreier, 1998). The disease model of same-sex desire also continues to be perpetuated through behavioural and biomedical research that attempts to identify the 'causes' of homosexuality or the 'physiological differences' between gay men or lesbians and heterosexuals (Wilton, 2000).

Given the above, it can seen how many gay people with sexual problems may be reluctant to be referred to psychosexual specialists because of the anticipated 'problematizing' of their sexual orientation or the perception that such services are not orientated to their needs (McNally and Adams, 2000).

Psychosexual problems

There is little empirical data available which details the type and prevalence of sexual problems in lesbians, gay men and bisexual men and women, although McNally and Adams (2000) and Crowley (2001a) provide a useful overview of some of the research that is available. One of the most commonly reported sexual difficulties in lesbian couples appears to be loss of sexual desire. This may reflect the tendency in society for women to be less often socially conditioned to initiate sex. Whilst, on average, lesbians may have sex less often than heterosexual women, research suggests they tend to have more frequent orgasms (both through masturbation and sex with partners) and greater sexual satisfaction than their heterosexual counterparts (Coleman et al., 1983). The sexual problems experienced by gay men are similar to those reported by heterosexual men, with erectile disorders being the most common problems reported. There is some research which suggests that gay men tend to experience more 'situational' rather than 'generalized' erectile problems and that such problems tend to occur more frequently in established relationships rather than casual sexual encounters (Paff, 1985). Gay men also appear to have less problems with premature ejaculation

and more difficulties with delayed/absent ejaculation than their heterosexual counterparts.

It is difficult to ascertain the type and prevalence of sexual problems
experienced by gay men, lesbians, and bisexual women and men, as
current classifications of psychosexual problems do not adequately
reflect the spectrum of sexual activities of gay men and lesbian women
(and, indeed, many heterosexual men and women). The type of sexual
activities commonly reported by gay men includes caressing, kissing,
mutual masturbation, oral sex and anal sex, although Bell (1999) notes
that up to a third of gay men probably choose not to practise anal sex on a
regular basis. Caressing, kissing, mutual masturbation and oral sex are
also common sexual acts reported by lesbians, with penetration using
fingers or possibly sex toys. Given this diversity of sexual activities, it is
clear that practitioners need to avoid making assumptions about the
sexual repertoire of individual gay, lesbian or bisexual patients. The
tendency to divide lesbian women and gay men in terms of being 'active'
or 'passive' on the basis of the role they are presumed to assume during
penetrative sexual acts is particularly unhelpful. As Coxon (1996)
observes, gay sex is not obsessively centred on penetration, and when
penetrative sexual acts do occur it is likely that many individuals will
assume both insertive and receptive roles during sex. The meaning and
significance of particular sexual behaviours will differ between bisexual,
lesbian and gay individuals as they do for heterosexuals.

The spectrum of possible precipitating and maintaining factors for
problems related to sexual function and satisfaction have been outlined in
Chapter 4, and may affect anyone, be they gay, lesbian, heterosexual or
bisexual. Gordon (1988), George (1993) and Simon (1996) suggest that
many sexual anxieties and difficulties for gay people, however, have their
origins in negative self-evaluations and unrealistic expectations about sex,
love and relationships. Gordon (1988) observes that working with gay
people with sexual difficulties requires an understanding not only of the
psychosomatic process but also an awareness of the role played by social
factors in creating a gay person's sexual identity.

All gay men and women will, whilst growing up, have internalized to
some degree what Gordon (1988, p. 249) terms 'the all-pervasive negative
messages about gay sexuality'. Cognitive dissonance can occur when an
individual believes that the sexual behaviour they engage in (or the sexual
identity that it may signify) is 'bad', 'unnatural' or 'immoral', and this may
be an important factor in the aetiology and maintenance of sexual
dysfunction (McNally and Adams, 2000). This has possibly been

exacerbated by the HIV epidemic as sex has become associated, either consciously or subconsciously, with the possibility of life-threatening illness (Odets, 1995). In some cases sexual desire may be present but the distress arising from internalized homophobia and heterosexism means that it is not (and perhaps is never) acted upon. Restricting attraction to unavailable people may also be a manifestation of internalized homophobia (Davies, 1996a). Internalized negative feelings and beliefs about same sex relationships can also mean that for some gay men and lesbians it may be harder to remain motivated to work on any sexual problems that may occur within their relationships (McNally and Adams, 2000).

Gay men and lesbian women are often defined by society solely in terms of their sexual behaviour. This form of homophobic reductionism leads to stereotyping (for example, that all gay men are always ready for sex, or have very high numbers of sexual partners) and can, if internalized, lead to people equating their sexual identity with their ability to 'perform' sexually (Paff, 1985). McNally and Adams (2000) observe, for example, that lesbians who are subject to the twin forces of homophobia and sexism can find themselves in a double bind where if they have a high sex drive they are not 'nice' women, but if they are not sexually active they are not really lesbians. Equating one's identity with sexual performance may also mean that there is a greater likelihood of gay people experiencing sexual problems that are the consequence of ' performance anxiety'. Shires and Miller (1998, p. 47), in a study of psychological factors associated with erectile dysfunction in heterosexual and gay men, observe that 'the crucial factor in the experience of erectile dysfunction seems to be a successful sexual performance in the context of a specifically characterized sexual identity, rather than being a simple question of sexual functioning *per se*'.

A further difficulty associated with equating sexual behaviour with sexuality is the splitting of sexual and emotional intimacy (George, 1993). Gordon (1988, p. 249), in a discusion of the impact of stereotyped gender role behaviour on relationships between gay men, remarks that 'Gay men are not reared to be gay, but they are socialized as males with the taboos on emotionality, sensuality and intimacy that this implies'. Consequently, some gay men are more likely to maintain self-esteem and sexual functioning by engaging only in sex where personal contact is minimal (NcNally and Adams, 2000). This can lead to difficulties, however, when they meet partners for whom sex and love are essentially bound together or when they seek to establish a long-term relationship. Furthermore, George (1993) observes that:

the expectation to be entirely happy and fulfilled via a sexual relationship is both pervasive and persuasive in society, for straight and non-heterosexual people. Many people seem to feel a burden of responsibility to be happy (in a one-to-one relationship) and successful (in sex), and hold notions which are bound to lead to disappointment and dissatisfaction. (George, 1993, p. 255)

Not only does this expectation exist, but lesbian, gay or bisexual individuals and couples must create their own models of relationships and do so in the face of negativity, ignorance and hostility. Faced with such negativity, some gay men and women develop a compensatory response, that is, a desire to become, or be seen as, the 'ideal' gay man, lesbian or same sex couple. This, in turn, may generate sexual problems either directly through performance anxiety, or indirectly by increasing stress in general and by making the recognition and acknowledgment of relationship problems more difficult (McNally and Adams, 2000). Simon (1996) suggests that gay and bisexual couples rarely recognize the 'pioneering element' of their relationships. Consequently, when relationship problems do arise they are often interpreted as confirmation of the old and erroneous adage that same-sex relationships are inevitably unsuccessful, rather than viewed as problems that anyone might expect to encounter at certain points in a relationship.

Key points of Chapter 7

- Being gay, lesbian or bisexual is neither a psychosexual problem, nor a manifestation of mental illness.
- Preconceived ideas about the sexual repertoire of individual gay men or lesbians are generally unhelpful, as is the assumption that the structures of same-sex relationships always mirror those of heterosexual relationships.
- There is relatively little attention given to the psychosexual problems of gay men, lesbians and bisexual men and women in psychosexual research and literature.
- Concerns about the possible 'pathologization' of their sexual orientation may make some gay men, lesbians and bisexuals reluctant to accept referral to specialist psychosexual counselling and therapy services.
- Practitioners working with non-heterosexual patients with psychosexual difficulties require not only an understanding of the psychosomatic process but also an awareness of the role of social factors in the creation, maintenance and expression of sexual difficulties.

Key reading

Bell, R. (1999) Homosexual men and women. ABC of sexual health. *British Medical Journal* **318**; 452–455.

McNally, I., Adams, N. (2000) Psychosexual issues. In: Neal, C., Davies, D. (eds). *Issues in Therapy with Lesbian, Gay, Bisexual and Transgender Clients*. Buckingham: Open University Press.

CHAPTER 8

Sexually transmitted infections

Introduction

Psychosexual problems are associated with genital and sexually transmitted infections in a number of different ways (Boag and Barton, 1993; Goldmeier, 2001). Patients who have psychosexual problems may change partners frequently in an attempt to resolve their difficulties, thereby putting themselves (and their partners) at increased risk of acquiring a sexually transmitted infection (or infections). Patients diagnosed with sexually transmitted infections may develop psychosexual difficulties, particularly if the infection is recurrent, recalcitrant or threatens fertility. Furthermore, the diagnosis of an infection in one or both partners can place great stress on a relationship, and on occasions, is used as an opportunity to vent sexual and relationship difficulties which may have existed for quite some time. Concerns about sexually transmitted infections, including HIV, may also be the 'presenting problem' for some patients with psychosexual problems (Crowley, 2001b).

Given the possible relationships between sexually transmitted infections and psychosexual problems described above, it is perhaps not surprising that practitioners who work within the specialty of genitourinary medicine may regularly encounter patients with psychosexual difficulties.

Genitourinary medicine/sexual health clinics

A network of genitourinary medicine clinics exists throughout the UK at which sexually transmitted infections are diagnosed and treated. Genitourinary medicine clinics are used by a wide demographic spectrum of the population. Data from a national survey in the UK revealed that 8.3% of men and 5.6% of women had attended a clinic in their lifetime

(Johnson et al., 1996). Staff working within genitourinary medicine departments are legally bound by The NHS Trusts and Primary Care Trusts (Sexually Transmitted Diseases) Directions, 2000) to keep confidential any information given by patients and any notes giving details of patients' sexual histories. In addition to this additional level of confidentiality, patients can refer themselves directly to any clinic in the UK and will be guaranteed access to practitioners who are used to talking about sex. For these reasons, Crowley (1997, p. 6) suggests that the genitourinary medicine clinic is the place where patients may bring with them 'the emotional baggage of sex gone wrong'. George (1993) observes that many people who use genitourinary medicine clinics are reluctant or unwilling to visit their own GP with their sexual concerns. This may be because they have engaged in acts or behaviours contrary to their own sexual mores, or because they feel that their lifestyle would elicit disapproval from others, or because they feel that their sex lives are too private or personal to discuss with their own GP. Sexual history-taking and genital examination are routine aspects of the process of care within the genitourinary medicine clinic, which in the context of the confidentiality and anonymity of the clinic environment, can enable patients to explore aspects of their sexuality previously hidden or denied (Nelson, 1999).

In one study of semi-structured interviews with 70 male and 70 female patients attending a clinic for sexually transmitted diseases, almost a quarter of men and two-fifths of women reported experiencing a sexual dysfunction (Catalan et al., 1981). All but one man and two women regarded their sexual dysfunction as a problem for which they would have liked help. In a more recent study of heterosexual patients attending a genitourinary medicine clinic, 20% of men and 8% of women were identified as having a sexual dysfunction (Goldmeier et al., 1997). In a survey of directors of genitourinary medicine services by Keane et al. (1997), 84% of respondents supported the provision of sexual dysfunction services within genitourinary medicine clinics, but only 42% provided such a service. Of those already providing such a service, Keane and colleagues (1997) concluded that the range of sexual problems most clinics were prepared to treat was impressive. The only patients with psychosexual difficulties commonly referred to other specialists in significant numbers were patients with sexual phobias or aversions, or patients with issues relating to sexual identity or gender dysphoria.

Nelson (1999) notes how ethical dilemmas involving confidentiality, the age of patients and patients' destructive behaviours (with regard to self or others) may generate conflicting feelings for practitioners working in this area. One of the central premises of psychosexual awareness is thinking about the difficult feelings practitioners experience in response to the patients they encounter is a way of understanding more about the patient's inner world. Nelson (1999) observes that in the context of genitourinary medicine clinics these responses often involve strong and sometimes very disturbing feelings that are far-removed from the ideals that practitioners may hold about 'the good nurse'.

Research suggests that up to a third of patients attending genitourinary clinics may have significant levels of psychological disturbance and distress (Ikkos et al., 1997). In an interesting paper, Coleman and Etchegoyen (1992) discuss how patients can use the confidentiality associated with genitourinary medicine clinics and turn it into secrecy as a means of denying the seriousness of their problems. As patients have often referred themselves to the clinic, information about previous medical, sexual and psychiatric problems is often restricted to the patient and controlled by the patient. GPs cannot be telephoned and old medical notes cannot be consulted. Coleman and Etchegoyen (1992) suggest that genitourinary medicine clinics, with their rigid boundaries between themselves and other professional systems within health care, are 'functionally isolated agencies' and this can resonate with the patient's isolation from their own feelings and emotional contact with people. They consider that the genitourinary medicine clinic lends itself 'to splitting between physical and psychological pain, and between sexuality and personal relationships' which, in turn, fits into the needs of some patients to keep distress 'secret'. Consequently, the extent of the patient's true difficulties may not be fully recognized. Coleman and Etchegoyen (1992) observe that help will be requested and accepted by these patients providing it does not address the real issues, such as broken patterns of relationships and emotional isolation. Thus, any attempt to address this, or referral to specialist mental health professionals, may be perceived as extremely threatening as 'the patient is faced with reconnection with unbearable feelings of pain and helplessness which may precipitate destructive acting out' (Coleman and Etchegoyen, 1992, p. 325).

The diagnosis of a sexually transmitted infection

The prompt detection and appropriate medical management of sexually transmitted infections has important implications for both the infected individual's health, in terms of reducing the likelihood of long-term morbidity, and public health, by reducing the onward transmission of infection. However, screening for sexually transmitted infections can have 'hidden costs' (Duncan and Hart, 1999).

Nelson (1999) suggests that:

> A person diagnosed with a sexually transmitted infection (STI) rarely feels that it is a simple medical matter. The amount of distress experienced by an individual will relate directly to their understanding of their sexuality, their feelings about the sexual acts involved and the context and relationships these are placed within. (Nelson, 1999, p. 116)

Nelson observes that the impact of any infection depends to some extent on the general psychological well-being of the individual concerned, but emotional responses to diagnosis may also vary considerably depending upon which infection or infections are diagnosed. In an analysis of the psychosocial impact of a diagnosis of *Chlamydia trachomatis* (the most common bacterial sexually transmitted infection in the UK) Duncan et al. (2001) identify a number of themes, including:

- The perception of stigma associated with sexually transmitted infection.
- Uncertainty about reproductive health after diagnosis.
- Anxieties about partners' reactions to the diagnosis of infection.

According to Duncan et al. (2001) anxieties about future reproductive morbidity are exacerbated by clinical uncertainty about the natural course of chlamydia and the difficulty of providing a prognosis in relation to reproductive effects. The diagnosis of chlamydia also introduces the possibility of infidelity into current relationships, although uncertainty about the duration of infection can be used to lessen the threat caused by diagnosis to a person's current sexual relationship. Interestingly, Duncan and colleagues (2001) observe that whilst emphasizing uncertainty about the duration of infection might lessen fears about infidelity, it could also increase a patient's anxieties about future reproductive morbidity.

The most frequently diagnosed viral sexually transmitted infection in the UK is human papillomavirus (HPV) infection which is the cause of ano-genital warts. Ano-genital warts are disfiguring and can have a number of psychosexual sequelae, including feelings of anger, anxiety and guilt. The diagnosis of warts can lead to impaired body image, loss of self-esteem and self-confidence (Dudley, 1995). Anxieties may revolve around future fertility, cancer risk and possible infectivity with regard to current or future sexual partners (Taylor et al., 1997; Maw et al., 1998). None of the currently available treatments will necessarily eradicate warts, eliminate

HPV and maintain clearance. Consequently, the duration of treatment is often long and recurrence rates are often 20–30% (Von Krogh et al., 2000). The psychological distress caused by genital warts is often the worst aspect of this disease. Unlike genital warts, genital herpes (caused by herpes simplex virus) can be a very painful condition. This combined with the lack of any treatment that will eradicate herpes simplex infection and the unpredictability of recurrence, has generated a reasonably large amount of research examining the psychosexual sequelae associated with the diagnosis of this infection. A review of this research by Shah and Button (1998) concludes that the possible psychological consequences of being diagnosed with herpes are numerous and vary in severity. They include depression, guilt and shame, low self-esteem and interpersonal difficulties. The most frequent responses, however, appear to be generalized anxiety (Derman, 1986; Lynch, 1988) and psychosexual problems (Shaw and Rosenfeld, 1987; Lynch, 1988). The possibility of infecting partners when asymptomatic also exists and although the risk of transmission resulting from 'sub-clinical viral shedding' is believed to be very low (Patel et al., 1997), this possibility may have an adverse effect on sexual relationships.

The presence of infections in the genital tract can result in pain and discomfort and may be a potential cause of dyspareunia. Recurring painful conditions may cause particular distress and disruption to the lives of those whom they affect. Irving et al. (1998) conclude that women with recurrent vaginal candidiasis were more likely to suffer clinical depression and reported that their candidiasis seriously interfered with their emotional and sexual relationships. Conditions closely associated with sexually transmitted infections, such as balanitis, prostatitis, epidydmo-orchitis, pelvic inflammatory disease and sexually acquired reactive arthritis, may all cause varying degrees of pain, discomfort and interference with a patient's sexual expression.

The diagnosis of a sexually transmitted infection often results in concerns about potential infidelity on the part of one or both partners. Successful treatment for infections such as chlamydia, gonorrhoea and syphilis requires the concurrent treatment of a patient's sexual partner or partners. The issue of informing sexual partners may cause some patients considerable concern and may be impeded by guilt, embarrassment, shame and fear. Disclosure can place relationships at risk, may lead to verbal abuse or physical violence, or the acquisition of a 'reputation' (Nelson, 1999). Patients diagnosed with infections that may recur, or may be transmitted when the patient is asymptomatic face particular dilemmas as to whether or not to inform any new sexual partner of their condition. As a consequence of this, some patients with conditions such as genital herpes may seek to avoid any new sexual relationship (Drob et al., 1985).

Sexually transmitted infections are not just medical or biological problems but also social phenomena and there is a long history of stigmatization associated with such infections (Brandt and Jones, 1999). Holgate and Longman (1998) report that all the participants in their study associated sexually transmitted infections with 'being dirty' and promiscuity, and consequently feared being judged by others. A large proportion of British men and women in a study by Maw et al. (1998) reported feeling disgust and shame at having genital warts. Many of the interviewees in the study by Duncan et al. (2001) had, before being diagnosed with chlamydia, perceived themselves as being relatively invulnerable to infection as they had associated sexually transmitted infections with stereotypical notions of contamination and delinquency. Many people associate sexual infections with certain 'types' of person, thereby creating a situation in which sexually transmitted infections are viewed as a condition of 'others' and therefore not personally relevant (Scoular et al., 2001). This phenomena has been perhaps most pronounced in recent times in relation to people diagnosed with HIV infection (Sontag, 1991; Gilmore and Somerville, 1994).

HIV infection

HIV links sex with life-threatening illness and consequently, the meanings attached to being HIV antibody positive are unmatched by any other screening test (Willis, 1992). Acknowledging that all medical screening tests confer both a social as well as biological status, Willis (1992) is of the opinion that being labelled 'HIV antibody positive' has greater implications for a person's identity than other medical diagnoses, 'akin to becoming a master status' (Willis, 1992, p. 174). This is also reflected in the observation of Waldby (1996, p. 113) that a positive HIV test result is not just a sign of seropositivity but also a sign of a 'transmission category'. The psychosocial consequences of being diagnosed as HIV antibody positive can be profound. From the beginning of the epidemic a label has been attached to HIV positive people reflective of the mode of likely acquisition. 'Innocent victims' is the term commonly used to describe infected children and haemophiliacs, whereas 'AIDS sufferers' and many more pejorative terms, are used to describe those whose infection is deemed to be the result of their presumed hedonistic (and stigmatized) 'lifestyle'. This social dynamic of 'victim blaming' can also be played out in the minds of people infected with HIV (Ratigan, 1997).

Catalan and Thornton (1999) observe that increases in anxiety and distress in people with HIV infection tend to occur at the time when an HIV diagnosis is initially made, when physical symptoms develop and when anti-retroviral treatments are commenced. Although the distress associated with being diagnosed as HIV positive, is usually self-limiting, Catalan and Thornton (1999, pp 189–190) suggest that 'the person's expectation of the result, how the information is given, and the nature of support available may have important effects'. The development of painful and debilitating conditions, such as Kaposi's sarcoma and peripheral neuropathy, and changes in body image associated with HIV and anti-retroviral treatments may also lead to depression and distress in affected individuals (Catalan et al., 1995; Firn, 1996; Catalan and Thornton, 1999). There are a large number of potential losses associated with HIV infection and HIV-related illness, including loss of certainty, loss of future hopes, loss of health, loss of body image, loss of control, relationship and sexual losses (Sherr and Green, 1996). Conversely, Catalan and Thornton (1999) observe that improvements in health and changes in health status that occur as the consequence of taking anti-retroviral treatments are also associated with a variety of difficulties and psychological problems. Such difficulties include adjusting to an extended life expectancy, uncertainty about the long-term efficacy and benefits of treatment, practical difficulties associated with adhering to treatment regimens and what Catalan and Thornton (1999, p. 194) describe as 'difficulties associated with normalization of emotional and sexual relationships'.

Sherr (1995) suggests that many of the psychological problems associated with HIV are linked to psychosexual issues, in particular relationship difficulties. Sherr (1995) notes that the diagnosis of HIV can cause relationship difficulties, and strain can also be placed on sexual relationships by alterations in sexual behaviours necessary to avoid the transmission of HIV and the need to negotiate openly behaviours which may have been accepted silently. The responses of partners and the strength of relationships prior to the diagnosis of HIV will all be relevant to the development of psychosexual difficulties (Catalan et al., 1995). A useful discussion of the impact of the diagnosis of HIV infection on partners and personal relationships is provided by Hedge (1999). George (1994) notes that the partners of individuals with HIV may cease to experience pleasure from sexual contact with their partners either because of worries about infection or more usually because of their partner's loss of interest and enthusiasm for sex. Reduced sex drive has commonly been observed in people infected with HIV and is a source of anguish for some. George (1994) reports that reduced sexual interest is particularly common in people who are newly diagnosed as they often feel sexually unacceptable, and lose interest and confidence in having sexual contact with either established or new sexual partners. Sometimes, however, the converse may be true as some people, particularly when newly diagnosed, may find themselves having sex compulsively as a means of proving to themselves that they are still sexually attractive or as a means of trying to overcome problems associated with sexual dysfunction. Catalan et al. (1995) observe that in the early stages of infection, the feelings of shock and distress associated with being diagnosed may lead to a reduced interest in sex and powerful feelings of guilt, contamination and fear of illness. Later, feelings of loneliness and the need for intimacy may conflict with concerns about infecting others, disfigurement and fear of death.

Sexual dysfunction is quite a common problem among people with HIV, particularly those who are symptomatic (Catalan et al., 1995; Catalan, 1999). The most frequently reported sexual problems are loss of interest in sex, erectile problems and ejaculatory problems (in particular, delayed ejaculation) in men, and loss of interest in sex, arousal difficulties and orgasmic dysfunction in women (Catalan and Thornton, 1999). Catalan et al. (1995) note that given the complexity of HIV, the causes of sexual dysfunction in HIV infection and disease are likely to arise from a combination of factors, including:

- Psychosexual reactions to HIV.
- Pre-existing sexual dysfunctions and associated disorders.
- HIV-related organic factors, for example, testicular and hormonal abnormalities, autonomic neuropathy.
- Iatrogenic causes, such as the side-effects of medication.

Thus, any assessment of sexual dysfunction in people with HIV needs to take account of the array of possible contributory factors before deciding what intervention would be appropriate (Catalan et al., 1995). Interventions designed to restore sexual function, will need also to address the issue of HIV prevention (that is preventing the onward transmission of HIV). Incorporating primary prevention into the delivery of treatment information, advice and support has become an even greater priority with the advent of anti-retroviral treatments (Summerside, 1999).

Sherr (1995) considers that HIV often brings many psychosexual problems to the fore. She notes that psychosexual issues not only surface in clinical work with people who know that they are HIV positive but also often emerge when counselling those who are contemplating having an HIV test. Choosing to have an HIV test is often the result of some personal crisis or has some sort of symbolic significance for the person concerned (Lupton et al., 1995a, 1995b; Nelson, 1999). George (1993) notes how AIDS counselling services have been used by some people to gain access to confidential support for psychosexual problems where the issue of HIV is not necessarily of great importance to them. The request for an HIV test may therefore act as a 'presenting problem' for other psychosexual issues.

The 'worried well'

Much has been written about the 'worried well', particularly in terms of HIV infection. The term has been used to refer to people who are worried about HIV or other sexually transmitted infections but who have not been tested and have no symptoms, but is more commonly used to refer to people who are excessively worried about HIV or another sexual infection, despite screening test results that are negative or objectively being at very little or no risk (Green and Kentish, 1996). George (1994) observes that the 'worried well' who present with excessive concerns about HIV infection or requesting HIV antibody testing may have underlying problems related to sexual orientation or sexual guilt over behaviours they regard as transgressing their own sexual mores. According to George (1994) sexual guilt may lead to communication difficulties with regular partners, problems related to sexual function (commonly loss or lack of pleasure or inadequate sexual arousal), phobic disorders where people 'punish' themselves with obsessive thoughts about HIV, or a combination of all three of these. Alternatively, pre-existing relationship or sexual problems may sometimes lead to people having sex with people other than their regular partner which, in turn, causes guilt, anxiety or fears about being infected with HIV. Sexual guilt may occur particularly in individuals who have been recently bereaved. Occasionally, the first sexual relationship after the loss of a long-term partner precipitates concerns about sexually transmitted infections. Attendance at a sexual health clinic for screening may enable individuals to share not only the guilt they may be experiencing but also some of the pain of their grief.

Most people who are excessively worried about having been infected with HIV or another sexual infection usually stop worrying when they receive the negative results of clinical and laboratory findings. Occasionally, however, individuals continue to have a persisting conviction that they are infected with HIV and often re-attend for further screening in the absence of very little or no new risk. These convictions are often fed by the presence of chronic anxiety-related symptoms, such as fatigue, intermittent diarrhoea, slight lymphadenopathy or slight weight loss, which are misinterpreted as signs of HIV-related disease. Individuals may also report obsessive–compulsive behaviours or ruminating thoughts about HIV infection and disease. Ruminating thoughts often focus on images of disease and death or routes of contagion – either situations which can lead on to the acquisition HIV or fears of transmitting the infection to others, particularly sexual partners and family members. The behavioural consequences of such thoughts include persistently checking the body for signs of infection (with pain and swelling often resulting from excessive palpation), scrutinizing partners for signs of infection and seeking further reassurance by searching out more information, contacting helplines, frequent medical consultations or repeat testing. The difficulty with such behaviours is that whilst they may bring transient relief and a concomitant reduction in anxiety, ultimately they reinforce morbid preoccupation and obsessive thoughts.

Catalan et al. (1995) suggest that such persistent concerns should be viewed as a symptom rather than a diagnosis. They note that irrational worries about HIV are sometimes seen in a wide range of different psychiatric disorders, including adjustment disorders, obsessional disorders, hypochondriasis or delusional in nature resulting from affective disorders such as major depression, mania or schizophrenia. Where persistent worries are the consequence of hypochondriasis (or health anxiety), obsessive or phobic disorder, the specialist management of such individuals is predominantly in line with the principles and practice of cognitive–behavioural therapy or cognitive therapy (see Wells, 1997; Miller et al., 1988). For delusional beliefs secondary to major depression or schizophrenic disorders, appropriate pharmacological interventions may be required (Catalan et al., 1995).

On occasions, some patients repeatedly attend genitourinary medicine clinics with somatic complaints for which there is no identifiable cause (Woolley, 1997). Such patients may have what Frost (1985) terms 'morbid bodily concern'. Frost (1985, p. 134) defines morbid bodily concerns as 'a state of anxious preoccupation with the possibility of illness, usually resulting from the misperception or misinterpretation of physical signs and symptoms'. The components of morbid bodily concern include nosophobia (a persistent unfounded fear of disease), psychogenic pain (as opposed to pain that is the consequence of altered physiology or functional changes resulting from psychosomatic reactions) and misperceptions of physical signs. In a study of 36 patients with 'somatic complaints' referred from a genitorurinary medicine clinic to a liaison psychiatric clinic for assessment, Frost (1985) examined 'illness behaviour' in terms of consultation behaviour, affective distress and psychological defensiveness. He found that the most obvious features of these patients' consultation behaviour were dissatisfaction and hostility. Affective distress – usually mild to moderate depression with varying degrees of anxiety – was evident in about half of the patients. Frost (1985) reports that it was impossible to engage the majority of patients over any psychological issues and he notes that patients tended to be defensive and hostile to the exploration of their personal life. He also reports that only a small number of the patients he initially interviewed returned for one or more sessions at the liaison psychiatry clinic and about half the group did not return to the genitourinary medicine clinic during the follow-up period.

Patients who attend repeatedly with persisting worries about HIV infection or other sexually transmitted infections, or somatic complaints for which no underlying physical pathology can be identified, can be demanding both in terms of the time and skill required to care for them. Nelson (1999) observes that these patients have a broad range of problems and suggests that by listening to their fears it may be possible for practitioners to help patients discover what function their worries are serving. It is unlikely that repeated screening or the provision of more information or reassurance, will bring patients anything other than transient relief from their anxieties. However, many patients experiencing such distress seem reluctant to engage in any exploration of possible psychological or relationship difficulties contributing to their problem. Trying to identify the 'causes' of patients' concerns by forcing them to explore the possible relationship between their feelings, thoughts and somatic symptoms or imposing one's own 'hypotheses' is usually counterproductive. This often results in a situation where patient and practitioner become locked in a 'battle of wills' which is not conducive to the creation of therapeutic space between practitioner and patient. Practitioners need to hold a position where they neither collude with the patient's definition of problem, nor dismiss the patient's own experience of his or her problem. At the same time practitioners need to find some way of acknowledging the anxiety and distress the patient is feeling and creating a therapeutic space. Although it is often counterproductive to insist that the patient views his or her problems as psychological in origin, it is often productive, to acknowledge, albeit tentatively, that the patient's worries and symptoms must be anxiety-provoking and stressful for him or her (Bor et al., 1998).

The term 'the worried well' is very much a misnomer as it fails to convey the anxiety and distress that many of those who are so labelled are actually experiencing. The care of such patients is challenging and sometimes isolating, particularly as patients may be reluctant to accept referral for more specialist psychological help. Practitioners need, therefore, to retain an awareness of the limitations to the help that they can offer.

Key points of Chapter 8

- A complex and, on occasions, synergistic relationship exists between sexually transmitted infection and psychosexual problems.
- The additional levels of confidentiality, open-access (ability to self-refer and to attend any clinic irrespective of area of residence) and focus on sexual matters means that genitourinary clinics are places where patients are more likely to bring their sexual concerns.
- Aspects of the 'process of care', such as taking a sexual history or performing a genital examination, may also make it more likely that patients disclose psychosexual difficulties or past traumatic experiences such as sexual assault or childhood sexual abuse.
- The 'meaning' and significance of screening tests for HIV and other sexually transmitted infections may vary greatly between patients.
- The emotional response of an individual to a diagnosis of a sexually transmitted infection depends on a number of factors. These may include which infection or infections are diagnosed, the degree of pain, discomfort and disruption to lifestyle associated with the condition, uncertainty about possible long-term effects on health and fertility, the anticipated reactions of partners and the perception of stigma.
- Many of the psychological problems associated with being HIV positive are linked to psychosexual issues and relationship difficulties.
- Sexual dysfunction is quite a common problem among people who are HIV positive. The causes of sexual dysfunction are likely to arise from a combination of factors, including psychosexual reactions to HIV, HIV-related organic factors and treatments used.

- HIV testing and counselling services may be used by certain patients who are seeking confidential support for psychosexual issues not necessarily related to HIV infection. This is often the 'hidden work' of many HIV testing services.
- Some patients who are worried about having HIV or another sexual infection, are not reassured by clinical and laboratory findings and re-attend for further examination and screening. Such individuals often report obsessive–compulsive behaviours or ruminating thoughts about the infection that preoccupies them. Offering reassurance or repeat screening seldom brings these patients anything other than transient relief from their anxieties.
- The genitals often provide a focus for psychosexual anxiety and distress, however, trying to 'force' an individual to see the link between emotions and symptoms for which no underlying pathology can be found, is likely to generate only greater defensiveness.

Key reading

Green, J. (2002) Psychological factors in sexually transmitted diseases. In: Miller, D., Green, J. (eds). *The Psychology of Sexual Health*, Oxford: Blackwell Science.

Nelson, S. (1999) Psychosexual issues in sexual health care. In: Weston, A. (ed.). *Sexually Transmitted Infections*. London: Nursing Times Books.

CHAPTER 9

Sexual assault and sexual abuse

Introduction

The experience of being sexually assaulted as an adult or sexually abused during childhood can make medical examination or intimate procedures, such as taking genital swabs or a cervical smear, intolerable. Even if undergoing such procedures is possible, patients' behaviour – both verbal and non-verbal – before, during and immediately after any such examination may communicate their distress, albeit indirectly, and may alert practitioners to the difficulty that they are experiencing. On occasions, however, extreme distress may 'come out of the blue', surprising or shocking both patient and practitioner. The practitioner's initial reaction when a patient discloses that she or he has been abused is extremely important. Hickerton (2001, p. 119) observes that 'a non-threatening, accepting and understanding attitude' will reduce any sense of abnormality the patient may be experiencing and will encourage the patient to talk. Often, practitioners who are uncertain how to respond may attempt to ignore the significance of what is being said or make a hasty referral to another professional or organization. Although referral to a psychologist or counsellor may be necessary for some patients who have been sexually assaulted or abused, it is important that patients do not feel immediately 'abandoned' by the person whom they have chosen to tell. Practitioners can feel under considerable pressure being both unsure how to respond and cognizant of other patients who are waiting to be seen. Practitioners who have had unwanted sexual experiences themselves can find working with patients who have been sexually abused or assaulted particularly difficult and may require access to additional support (Hardman et al., 1998).

Care for the victims of sexual assault

Some patients may present to health services soon after being sexually assaulted in order to eliminate the possibility of having acquired a sexual infection. For other patients, certain aspects of the process of care, such as giving a sexual history or undergoing a genital examination, can trigger memories of previous traumatic sexual experiences (Nelson, 1999). Sexual abuse and assault both result in trauma, although the extent and duration of the traumatic after-effects of such experiences will be mediated by a number of factors, including age at which abuse occurred, the duration of any assault or abuse, the relationship of the patient to the perpetrator and whether the patient has been assaulted on more than one occasion (Hennebry, 1998; Nelson, 1999; Petrak, 2002).

The Sexual Offences Act (1994) defines rape as 'vaginal penetration of a woman, or anal penetration of a person of either gender without their consent, or with willful disregard to their consent'. Moore (1998) notes that:

> For most women, rape represents many different types of assault that happen simultaneously: on their sense of control over their own life and on their trustful assumptions about others and their safety in the world. It is also a devastating intrusion of their personal space. (Moore, 1998, p. 53)

Rape is generally under-reported. Moore (1998) notes that the ordeal of having to undergo a medical examination is often enough to deter many women from reporting the crime, although the fear of further pain and humiliation associated with the judicial process deters many others from reporting attacks. Male rape also seems to be rarely reported to the police. The act of forced anal penetration in men often stimulates the prostate gland resulting in involuntary penile erection and ejaculation. A lack of awareness of this fact and fears about how this subsequently may be used and reported often deters the reporting of male rape (Rogers, 1999; Cybulska and Forster, 2001). It is also important for practitioners working with refugees and asylum seekers to be aware that rape is often one aspect of the torture and organized violence that some refugees may have experienced (Burnett and Peel, 2001).

Hennebry (1998) notes that people who are raped often feel dirty and blame themselves for their ordeal. Practitioners need to ensure that no act or intimation on their part, reinforces this perception. Hennebry (1998) writes that it is important to reiterate to a patient who has been raped that she or he did the right thing. Initial support for victims of sexual assault should reinforce the victim's sense of autonomy and freedom to choose the type of help she or he wants. This is important as many people who are sexually assaulted often experience feelings of helplessness and of things being out of their control. If the patient wishes to report the incident to the police he or she should be advised that a forensic examination (which can be useful in terms of evidence collection up to seven days after the assault) should be performed prior to any other medical examination. It is also important that patients are aware that it is exceptional for the identification of a sexually transmitted infection to be used as evidence in court as prior acquisition would have to be excluded. Indeed, disclosing the diagnosis of such an infection in court may sometimes harm rather than help a survivor's case, although conversely the finding of a sexually transmitted infection may influence the level of criminal injuries compensation (Lacey, 1999).

Recent national guidelines (Lacey, 1999) suggest that full screening for sexually transmitted infections should be offered to adults who have been raped, as research does suggest that there is a small but significant incidence of the acquisition of a sexually transmitted infection resulting from rape. Not all infections are detectable immediately following a sexual act and some tests may need to be repeated 2 to 12 weeks after the sexual assault (Hedge, 2002). A discussion about HIV infection should also be part of any initial consultation. It should be noted that, although HIV seroconversion has followed sexual assault, available research suggests that the risk of HIV acquisition following heterosexual assault in the UK is low. The anxieties of patients who have been sexually assaulted by previous or current sexual partners may be very different from those who have been sexually assaulted by strangers. Post-exposure prophylaxis (often referred to as PEP) using anti-HIV drugs after sexual exposure is still controversial (King, 1998; Hayter, 1999), although some clinics do provide PEP for people who have been exposed to HIV through sex on a case-by-case basis (King, 1998). If PEP is to be given it is recommended that it should start no later than 72 hours after a 'high-risk' sexual exposure and that patients need to be aware of the unproven efficacy and potential toxicity of the treatment (Lacey, 1999).

It is recommended that hepatitis B vaccine should be offered to all victims of sexual assault. In situations where patients may not re-attend, or are unable to tolerate the distress of an examination, or require an intrauterine contraceptive device to be inserted as emergency contraception, prophylactic antimicrobial treatment that would cover both chlamydia and gonorrhoea may also be offered. Finally, if there is a risk of pregnancy post-coital contraception in the form of either hormonal treatment (which can be given up to 72 hours after the assault) or an intrauterine contraceptive device should be offered.

Nelson (1999) observes that many people who have been sexually assaulted attend for screening soon after the attack on them has occurred, and despite their distress at this time only a few wish to discuss what has happened. Indeed, a recent review of available research suggests that routine 'debriefing' (a single-session intervention soon after a traumatic event) is not generally helpful in preventing later post-traumatic disorders (Department of Health, 2001b). Nelson (1999) does suggest, however, that victims of sexual assault may benefit from being given leaflets that contain information about dealing with some of the possible manifestations of post-trauma stress, such as nightmares, panic attacks or having difficulties with sleeping and eating. After the shock of being sexually assaulted, many survivors experience feelings of depression, anxiety, guilt, anger and loss. Moore (1998) suggests that survivors of rape can be expected to work through a grieving process in the same way as a person who has suffered a bereavement. Hennebry (1998) notes that other difficulties survivors of sexual assault may experience include:

• Difficulties leaving the house/difficulties going to work.
• Suicidal ideation.
• Problems related to alcohol and drug misuse.
• Relationship difficulties.
• Psychosexual problems.

Problems may be exacerbated by the response the survivor of sexual assault receives from others, such as partners, family, friends and the criminal justice system (*see* Moore, 1998). Blame is often directed towards the survivors of sexual assault and it is not unusual for patients to report that friends and family members are both shocked and revolted (Hennebry, 1998). Hennebry (1998) also observes that a number of factors may compound the anger, grief or isolation experienced by a survivor of a sexual assault, including:

• Previous experience of being sexually assaulted.
• The experience of childhood sexual abuse.
• Being gay or lesbian.
• Experiencing a crisis about their sexuality at the time of the assault.
• Being a prostitute.
• Male rape.

Where a survivor of sexual assault does present with post-traumatic stress disorder, referral for psychological therapy is indicated (see Lee, 2002; Petrak and Hedge, 2002). Currently, there is evidence that patients with post-traumatic stress disorder can receive substantial help from psychological therapy, particularly therapy that utilizes cognitive behavioural methods (Department of Health, 2001b).

The effect of childhood sexual abuse on sexual identity in adult life

Doyle (1998) observes that it is difficult to state with any authority what the consequences of childhood sexual abuse are. The term 'childhood sexual abuse' can cover a wide range of abusive experiences and Doyle (1998) suggests that:

> The exact nature and duration of the act are important, along with the use of threats, violence and coercion. In addition, details of the victim and the perpetrator combine to make each case unique. The victim's age and developmental stage, their premorbid personality and relationships with the abusers are key points, as are the abuser's age and gender (Doyle, 1998, p. 109)

Research by Bulik et al. (2001) suggests that survivors of childhood sexual abuse may be at greater risk of subsequent psychiatric disorders if:

- The abuse involved attempted or completed sexual intercourse.
- Threat or force was used by the perpetrator.
- The abuse was perpetrated by a relative.
- The victim received a negative response from someone in whom he or she confided.

Doyle (1998) notes that a distinction is often made between abuse that occurs between family members (intrafamilial) and sexual abuse that occurs where the perpetrator is outside the family (extrafamilial). Intrafamilial sexual abuse tends to be more common than extrafamilial child sexual abuse. Doyle (1998) also notes that the breach of trust associated with intrafamilial childhood sexual abuse makes disclosure more problematic in that it poses a threat to the continued existence of the family. By contrast, the disclosure of extrafamilial sexual abuse, providing it is believed, often results in the family remaining united and being supportive. Consequently, extrafamilial sexual abuse tends to present earlier than sexual abuse that occurs within a family. Additionally, when working with the victims of intrafamilial sexual abuse, it is often difficult to separate the consequences of being sexually abused from the consequences of being in a dysfunctional family. As Mullen et al. (1994) observe, sexual abuse, physical abuse and emotional abuse are often found together.

McCarthy (1990) suggests that there are three levels of 'victimization' associated with sexual traumas such as childhood sexual abuse. These are: the incident itself; how the experience is dealt with; and the manner in which it is integrated into a person's sexual self-esteem. McCarthy (1990) suggests that how the incident is dealt with and how it is integrated into an individual's sexual self-esteem often cause more trauma than the actual incident. He notes:

> This is especially true when the person keeps the incident secret, resulting in guilt and self-blame. Over time the secret becomes more distorted and powerful. Sexual expression causes additional guilt and pain. Sexuality is viewed as a negative part of life. (McCarthy, 1990, p. 143)

Finkelhor and Browne (1985) postulate four 'traumagenic dynamics' or trauma-causing factors associated with, although not unique to, childhood sexual abuse which may alter the child's cognitive and emotional orientation to the world, and in so doing adversely affect the normal development of autonomy, self-esteem and sexuality. These traumagenic dynamics are:

• Traumatic sexualization.
• Betrayal.
• Stigmatization.
• Powerlessness.

Traumatic sexualization

This refers to the process whereby an individual's sexuality is shaped 'in a developmentally inappropriate and interpersonally dysfunctional fashion as a result of sexual abuse' (Finkelhor and Browne, 1985, p. 531). This process can occur when a child is 'rewarded' for his or her sexual behaviour by the perpetrator with attention, affection, favours or gifts. Consequently, a child learns to use his or her sexual behaviour to manipulate others as a means to satisfying a variety of developmentally appropriate needs. Traumatic sexualization may also occur when certain parts of a child's anatomy are 'fetishized' and given a distorted importance and meaning, through the misconceptions about sexual behaviour and mores that are acquired from the perpetrator, and when frightening memories and events become associated in a child's mind with sexual activity. Finkelhor and Browne (1985) suggest that experiences in which the perpetrator attempts to evoke a sexual response in the child are probably more traumagenic than those where no such enticement occurs.

Betrayal

Refers to the discovery by a child that someone on whom he or she depends has caused them harm. Betrayal may occur not only at the hands of the perpetrator but also as a result of not being believed by those in whom the child confides, or by other family members who are colluding with the perpetrator of the sexual abuse. Doyle (1998) remarks that how the child's mother reacts in cases of intrafamilial sexual abuse appears to be particularly important. He notes that the mother may be faced with a choice – to stay with her abusing partner and reject her child, or to reject her partner and support her child. Doyle (1998, p. 108) observes 'thus the mother's own emotional needs enter the equation, and surely the saddest cases are when an abused child is further traumatized by maternal rejection'.

Stigmatization

Refers to the negative connotations communicated to the child about his or her experiences that become incorporated into the child's self-image. This may come directly from the perpetrator who further demeans and 'blames' the child for the activity or more indirectly through pressure exerted by the perpetrator on the child to 'keep a secret', thereby conveying powerful messages about guilt, shame and a sense of being 'different'. This may be further reinforced by the attitudes the child hears or infers from other people, especially 'significant others', and by adverse reactions to any disclosure of being abused.

Powerlessness

Finkelhor and Browne (1985, p. 532) define powerlessness as 'the process in which the child's will, desires, and sense of efficacy are continually contravened'. They postulate that powerlessness occurs in sexual abuse when a child's territory and body are repeatedly invaded against the child's will and is further exacerbated when the child's attempts to halt the abuse are frustrated.

Doyle (1998) observes that, in general, guilt and low self-esteem are prominent in children who are, or have been, sexually abused. Changes may also occur in a child's behaviour. Behaviours that may be associated with the experience of sexual abuse include 'sexualized' behaviour, anti-social behaviours, deliberate self-harm, eating disorders, running away from home, reverting back to less mature ways of behaving and the presentation of psychosomatic symptoms. Doyle (1998) also describes an 'accommodation syndrome' whereby abused children display no symptoms of their abuse. Doyle (1998, p. 108) notes that 'these cases can come to light when the child is surprised to learn that its peers are not sexually active and that the acts they have been involved in are not a normal part of childhood'.

A number of researchers have investigated whether there is a relationship between childhood sexual abuse and difficulties in adult social, interpersonal and sexual functioning and mental illness. The findings of many of these studies need to be interpreted cautiously owing to a number of methodological 'weaknesses', such as being retrospective, the use of unvalidated self-reports and biased sampling (Doyle, 1998). Mullen et al. (1994) who conducted research into the effects of childhood sexual abuse (CSA) on the social, interpersonal and sexual function of women living in New Zealand, report that:

> CSA would appear to be most disruptive of the attitudes to sexual activity and the attributions the individual makes to their own sexuality. Sexuality and sexual behaviour have, for a significant proportion of the CSA group become areas of uncertainty and difficulty rather than satisfaction. There was a clear overlap between sexual difficulties and wider relationship problems. In practice the CSA group was more prone to experience a disruption of intimacy, part of which was sexual and part the caring and emotional closeness of the relationships. (Mullen et al., 1994, p. 44)

It would be a mistake to assume that sexual, interpersonal and social difficulties are an inevitable outcome of sexual abuse for every person who has experienced this violation during childhood. A number of studies do indicate that patients who use psychiatric services are more likely to have a history of sexual abuse (Wurr and Partridge, 1997; Coxell et al., 1999). Although it cannot be concluded that the psychological problems of these patients are the direct result of their experiences of childhood abuse, the experience of childhood sexual abuse is often viewed as a 'vulnerability factor' for developing mental health problems in later life (Jehu, 1991; Lab, 2000).

Responding to the disclosure of childhood sexual abuse

Patients may disclose their experience of childhood sexual abuse in a number of ways. Disclosure may occur when a sexual history is being taken, or it may happen – sometimes dramatically – when intimate procedures are being carried out. Crises or life-changing events in a person's life, including ill-health that threaten a person's sexual identity, may also trigger patients to confide in practitioners. Selby (2001) notes that the disclosure of sexual abuse as a child may also come through the presentation of a psychosexual anxiety or difficulty and that patients may seek frequent consultations and may have tried to drop several hints about their emotional distress before any disclosure is made. Selby (2001) acknowledges that most practitioners to whom such disclosures are made, will be 'working from a position of ignorance' and will be left feeling shocked and confused as to how best to help. Selby (2001) cautions that it is important to keep normal responses of shock, distress, anger and condemnation to oneself as the patient discloses his or her experiences. Butler and Joyce (1998), discussing the work of counsellors with survivors of childhood sexual abuse, make some observations that may be pertinent to nurses caring for patients who have been sexually abused. They observe that:

> The work can rouse many uncomfortable feelings in the counsellor – longing to repair the irreparable, deep discomfort with the sense of voyeurism and sexual arousal that can accompany the work, despair at the bleak picture of man's cruelty and indifference to suffering that the accounts of the survivors can paint. (Butler and Joyce, 1998, p. 159)

Butler and Joyce (1998, p. 159) also outline a number of steps that people take in 'the journey from being a victim to being a survivor', these include:

- Telling their story.
- Working out who is responsible for the abuse.
- Experiencing the feelings associated with their abuse safely.
- Making sense of what has happened to them.
- Getting on with life.

Where patients disclose for the first time their experience of childhood sexual abuse, simply having the opportunity to tell their story is significant in itself. Selby (2001) remarks that the feelings that accompany sexual abuse include helplessness, violation, powerlessness, betrayal, guilt and, sometimes, sexual excitement. Such feelings may be difficult for practitioners to 'hear', as may the inability of some survivors to blame their abusers for what has happened. Some patients may require longer-term support or more intensive and specialized help than a nurse can offer. All patients should be made aware of the existence of any local self-help or specialist counselling organizations. Those patients with a high degree of disturbance in their social, interpersonal and sexual functioning may require referral to a psychologist or psychotherapist who specializes in working with patients who have been sexually abused as children (see Kennerley, 2002).

When caring for patients who have been sexually abused there are a number of issues which practitioners need to keep in mind. The first of these is described by Butler and Joyce (1998, pp 159–160) and is a relationship pattern that is commonly encountered where abuse has occurred. The dynamic of the relationship can be described thus. The practitioner views the patient as a 'victim' to be 'rescued'. The practitioner's perception of him- or herself as a 'rescuer' is reinforced by the patient's choice of that practitioner as a person in whom they confide their experience of abuse. In response to these feelings, the practitioner starts to work in ways that are different from his or her pattern of work with other patients. Examples of this may include offering more consultations than usual, extending consultations, meeting the patient outside of the clinical context or not referring the patient to more specialist sources of help and support when this is indicated. This increasingly exclusive attention generates from the patient requests for further help and support leading the practitioner soon to feel that he or she is the 'victim' of a demanding, insistent and 'persecuting' patient. Consequently, the practitioner looks for some way to be 'rescued' from this relationship. This usually involves seeking the advice of colleagues, clinical supervisors or line-managers, who inevitably advise returning the relationship to that which is indicative of usual clinical work. In response to this change in 'the rules of engagement' the patient may abruptly and angrily end the relationship and is left feeling a victim again. The practitioner is left with feelings of having failed his or her patient and of being unsympathetically treated by his or her colleagues, supervisor or manager.

A second difficulty can occur when practitioners seek to impose their 'own agenda' about childhood sexual abuse on a patient. The most extreme example of this occurs when a practitioner seeks to persuade, either directly or indirectly, a patient that his or her psychosexual or relationship difficulties are the consequence of previous sexual abuse as a child that has been 'forgotten' or 'repressed'. Where previous abuse is suspected, it may be appropriate to 'enquire gently' whether the patient has been abused in the past (Selby, 2001, p. 92) or more generally, as McCarthy (1990, p. 143) suggests, to ask what has been the most negative or traumatic sexual experience in a patient's life. If a patient does confirm that he or she has been sexually abused as a child, it would be wrong to try to 'force' the patient to make a connection between this and the current psychosexual anxieties or difficulties he or she is experiencing. This reflects the practitioner's desire to find an 'answer' to the patient's difficulties and is the opposite of creating a therapeutic space between practitioner and patient which may enable patients to discover the links between their emotions and their current sexual problems. Attributing a patient's sexual anxieties and distress automatically to childhood sexual abuse may mean that other causes for these feelings remain unaddressed. It may also convey the practitioner's conviction or judgement that all survivors of childhood sexual abuse are destined to develop sexual and relationship difficulties. As Mullen et al. (1994, p. 45) observe, although those who report childhood sexual abuse are more likely to experience a range of sexual, interpersonal and social difficulties in adult life, 'abuse is not destiny'.

Conversely, a patient's disclosure of being sexually abused as a child should never go unacknowledged. Failure to acknowledge a patient's disclosure colludes with the perpetrators of such abuse and violates the duty of care owed to the patient. It may also convey that this issue is too painful or too taboo to be discussed openly. In caring for patients who have been abused, it is necessary, however, for practitioners to listen to the significance and meaning such experiences have for each individual patient, rather than making assumptions based on what they have read or encountered previously in either their personal lives or clinical practice.

Key points of Chapter 9

- The experience of sexual assault as an adult and sexual abuse during childhood can make intimate procedures, such as genital/pelvic/rectal examination or taking genital swabs and samples, extremely distressing or intolerable.
- The practitioner's initial reaction to any disclosure of sexual abuse or assault is extremely important.

- Both sexual abuse and sexual assault are traumatic experiences, although the extent and duration of the traumatic after-effects of these experiences will be mediated by a number of factors, including the age at which abuse occurred, the duration of any assault or abuse, the relationship of the patient to the perpetrator and whether the patient has previously been sexually assaulted.
- Initial support for the survivors of sexual assault and abuse include listening to the patient's story, keeping one's own feelings of shock, anger and distress to oneself and ensuring that the patient retains the freedom to decide what help he or she requires.
- Routine 'debriefing' shortly after a traumatic event is unlikely to help prevent post-traumatic stress disorder, although the provision of written information that identifies some of the potential emotional responses following sexual assault and sources of help and support, may be helpful.
- The experience of childhood sexual abuse does not automatically mean that a person will experience interpersonal and sexual difficulties later in life, although for many people who have been sexually abused during childhood, sexuality and sexual behaviour may be areas of uncertainty and difficulty rather than satisfaction and pleasure.

Key reading

Berry, M. (1997) Coming to terms with sexual abuse. *British Journal of Sexual Medicine* **24**, 3, 10–13.

Coxell, A.W., King, M.B. (2002) Gender, sexual orientation and sexual assault. In: Petrak, J. Hedge, B. (eds) *The Trauma of Sexual Assault*, Chichester: John Wiley & Sons Ltd.

CHAPTER 10

Sexual variations and issues relating to gender identity

Introduction

Although it is relatively rare that practitioners working in general health care settings will encounter patients presenting with anxieties or distress relating to sexually variant behaviours or gender identity problems, it is important that practitioners do have some knowledge of what help and support can be offered to such patients. Encountering and staying alongside such patients in clinical practice inevitably causes many practitioners to re-examine their own sexualities and assumptions about normality and, in so doing, requires them to confront some of their own confusions, insecurities and fears.

The psychosexual issues addressed in this chapter include paraphilias, transvestism and transsexualism. All of these issues are framed to varying degrees in Western society by social attitudes, the law and notions of pathology and normality. When encountering patients with these psychosexual issues, it can be particularly difficult to elude the reductionism of a label or diagnostic category and to remain aware of the individual as a whole person. Like all patients who are anxious or distressed, such patients require someone who is prepared to listen to their concerns.

Sexual variations or paraphilias

The terms 'paraphilia' or 'sexual variations' are used by clinicians and researchers to refer to sexual desires and behaviours that are considered 'atypical' (De Silva, 1999). As always with behaviour, however, what is atypical or unusual varies between cultures and over time, therefore any definition of 'normality' is often arbitrary and consequently problematic in its application. Watson and Davies (1997) offer the following observation:

most paraphilias involve behaviours that play a small part in usual adult lovemaking – for example, exposing, sexual looking, dominating, submitting, dressing up, and regard for particular objects. In a paraphilia, however, such behaviour becomes the erotic end in itself. (Watson and Davies, 1977, p. 242)

The essential features of a paraphilia, as outlined in the DSM-IV (APA, 1995, p. 536), are 'recurrent, intense sexually arousing fantasies, sexual urges, or behaviours generally involving 1) nonhuman objects, 2) the suffering or humiliation of one's partner, or 3) children or other nonconsenting persons, that normally occur over a period of 6 months'. For some individuals, paraphiliac fantasies or stimuli are always included in sexual activity, whereas for others paraphiliac preferences only occur episodically, such as at times of extreme stress. At other times, the person is able to become sexually aroused and engage in sexual activity without paraphiliac stimuli.

Examples of paraphilias include:

- Exhibitionism: gaining sexual pleasure and excitement from exposing one's genitals to others, usually strangers. Exposure of the genitals is sometimes accompanied by masturbation.
- Fetishism: recurrent sexual arousal or behaviour focused on the use or presence of inanimate objects, such as items of clothing, footwear, etc.
- Paedophilia: sexual excitement or sexual activity involving prepubescent children. De Silva (1999) states that to meet the diagnostic criteria for paedophilia, a person must be at least 16 years old and at least five years older than his or her victim(s). De Silva (1999, p. 654) also observes that 'most paedophiles are heterosexual and are often married with their own children, although they commonly have marital or sexual difficulties or problems with alcohol. Eighty per cent have a history of childhood sexual abuse'.
- Sexual sadism: gaining sexual enjoyment and satisfaction from inflicting pain on others.
- Sexual masochism: deriving sexual pleasure or satisfaction from incurring pain or humiliation.
- Voyeurism: the observation of unsuspecting individuals who are naked, undressing or engaging in sexual activity.
- Frotteurism: touching and rubbing one's genitals against a nonconsenting person.

Other sexual variations include:

- Zoophilia or bestiality: sexual desire for animals.
- Necrophilia: sexual desire for corpses.
- Urophilia: sexual arousal from contact with urine.
- Coprophilia: sexual arousal from contact with faeces.

The most common presenting problems in clinics that specialize in the treatment of paraphilias are paedophilia, voyeurism and exhibitionism. Many individuals have more than one paraphilia. Furthermore, although the diagnostic categorization of paraphilias is based on the characteristic paraphiliac focus, it does not necessarily convey the significance or meaning of these sexual interests or acts for the individuals concerned. As always, in labelling or categorizing aspects of patient's sexuality, there is a danger that the patient will cease to be viewed as a whole person.

Practitioners working in general health care settings are likely to encounter patients presenting with paraphilias only if their paraphilia is causing them or their partners distress or anxiety, or if they are experiencing another health or sexual problem that is secondary to paraphiliac activity. Headon (1998) considers that it is important that the element of fear and distress patients may feel about their sexuality is recognized and listened to. However, patients presenting with anxiety or distress associated with paraphilias are also likely to evoke strong feelings in many practitioners, some of which may be shared by the patient. Headon (1998) also notes that:

> scientific objectivity cannot conceal a considerable fearfulness about what these paraphilias are, or what they mean. This fear is experienced also by the clients presenting with paraphilias or their sexual partners. (Headon, 1998, p. 195)

Awareness of this is important; Headon (1998) suggests that one of the basic fears associated with paraphilias concerns the potential for loss of control and the fear that behaviours might very easily get out of hand unless action is taken to prevent this. Certain paraphiliac activities are illegal and the disclosure of such activities by a patient requires practitioners to consider the ethical, professional and legal implications of their response (see Chapter 2). Practitioners need to be aware that many people presenting with paraphilias will be suffering from fears around both having and losing control (Headon, 1998).

Treatment for paraphilias

The assessment and treatment of paraphilias is a specialist matter, although the provision of specialist services tends to be erratic (Watson and Davies, 1997). Interventions used to treat paraphilias have included psychological methods such as 'orgasmic reconditioning', aversion therapy and group therapy, and pharmacological treatment involving the use of drugs, such as medroxyprogestrone acetate and cyproterone acetate, to reduce sex drive and hence paraphiliac behaviours. Wylie (1998) reports that there is also some evidence that the selective serotonin re-uptake inhibitor group of drugs may also be of some benefit in the treatment of paraphilias such as exhibitionism and voyeurism.

Although pharmacological treatment may eliminate the performance of paraphiliac activities, it does not always remove troublesome desires, and certain psychological 'treatments', such as aversive reconditioning by use of electric shocks and nausea-creating drugs, are viewed by many as being ineffective in the long-term and abusive (Headon, 1998).

De Silva (1999) writes that if the goal of treatment is to eliminate paraphiliac behaviour, it needs to be recognized that success may be limited as treatment approaches tend merely to suppress rather than eradicate paraphiliac behaviours. An alternative treatment aim to elimination is incorporation, that is, to incorporate the paraphilia in a controlled way into the person's sexual repertoire. Although this approach is not possible for certain sexual variations, such as paedophilia, De Silva (1999) considers that it is an approach that may benefit people whose partners are distressed by the prominence of the paraphilia in their sexual relationship.

Transvestism

The ICD-10 (WHO, 1992) describes two forms of transvestism: 'fetishistic transvestism' and 'dual role-transvestism'. Fetishistic transvestism refers to sexual arousal associated with wearing articles of clothing of the opposite sex. It may be considered an example of a paraphiliac behaviour in that once orgasm has occurred and sexual arousal has diminished, the individual normally wishes to remove these articles of clothing. By contrast, in dual role transvestism, there is no sexual motivation for cross-dressing. The individual who is a dual role transvestite wears clothes of the opposite sex in order to experience temporary membership of the opposite sex, although usually has no wish for any permanent form of gender reassignment. Webster (2001) observes that most transvestites are heterosexual men. She notes that there is now a reasonably extensive support network, begun by the Beaumont Society, of social organizations and voluntary groups for dual-role transvestites and their partners as well as a small commercial industry serving the needs of individuals who cross-dress.

Webster (2001) observes that attempts at eradicating cross-dressing by any form of treatment are usually futile. Instead she suggests that 'a more helpful approach is to de-pathologize the situation and encourage the patient to integrate the cross-dressing safely, comfortably and creatively into his life' (Webster, 2001, p. 176). Webster (2001) acknowledges, however, that this in part is dependent on an individual's home situation and the reaction of partners.

Gender identity

Gender development starts from the moment of conception. Consequently, certain gender problems may be congenital. Certain genetic conditions, such as congenital adrenal hyperplasia or androgen insensitivity syndrome, may result in the masculinization of genetically female infants (congenital adrenal hyperplasia) and the feminization of genetically male infants (androgen insensitivity syndrome). The extent of these processes of feminization and masculinization will vary between children. Some children will be born with ambiguous genitalia and decisions will need to be made as to the sex of rearing and whether surgery to alter the appearance of the genitalia is desirable. The decision about which sex a child will be reared as requires full discussion between clinicians and parents. In a recent article titled 'Surgery for intersex', Creighton (2001) observes that clinicians tend to choose the gender that carries the best prognosis for reproductive and sexual function and for which the genitalia can be made to look most normal. If surgery is required, it is usually performed as soon as possible. The focus of genital surgery is on the cosmetic appearance of the genitals rather than later sexual function, and the justification for such intervention is often the assumption that a child must have unambiguous genitals in order to achieve a stable gender identity (Creighton and Minto, 2001). However, Creighton (2001) writes that every aspect of this area is currently under review, including diagnostic techniques, and the timing and nature of treatments, including surgery. Creighton (2001) refers to an increasing body of knowledge which suggests that many adults are unhappy and feel mutilated by the surgery performed on them as children and notes that the centrality of genital surgery in facilitating successful psychosocial adjustment is now being questioned. Creighton (2001) also reports that some prominent intersex support groups recommend that no surgery should be performed unless absolutely necessary, and that some commentators advocate an even more radical approach, namely that there should be no attempt to allocate an intersex child to male or female gender but that a third gender should be recognized.

The masculinization and feminization of some children means that some genetically male infants will be identified and reared as females from birth and some genetically female infants will be identified and reared as males from birth. The genetic sex of such children may only become apparent later in their development, sometimes as a result of a failure to develop secondary sexual characteristics of their allocated gender. This indicates that social factors have a strong influence on the gender identity (the sense of oneself as being male or female) of such children. Golombok and Fivush (1998) observe that:

> Biological males with complete androgen insensitivity syndrome who look female at birth and who are raised as girls can develop female gender identity, and biological females with congenital adrenal hyperplasia who look like boys and who are treated as boys can develop male gender identity – in spite of incongruent sex chromosomes, gonads, hormones and internal reproductive organs! The most important factor in determining gender identity seems to be the sex to which the infant is assigned and reared. (Golombok and Fivush, 1998, p. 32)

Transsexualism

Transsexualism, sometimes referred to as 'gender dysphoria' or 'gender identity disorder' (GID), is a term (and diagnosis) used to describe individuals who show a strong and persistent cross-gender identity. This is usually accompanied by a persistent discomfort with their anatomical sex and feelings that the gender roles associated with their sex are inappropriate (Cohen-Kettenis and Gooren, 1999). In clinical practice, practitioners may encounter people who are affected by issues relating to gender identity in a number of different contexts. Individuals may present with difficulties directly associated with transsexualism in themselves or a partner. Practitioners may be involved in the care of patients undergoing gender reassignment surgery, or more commonly, may meet patients who completed gender reassignment surgery but have other health needs.

Finally, practitioners may be working alongside colleagues who are transsexuals.

Much of the medical literature on transsexualism is dominated by the issues involved in the physical reassignment of gender, and indeed, for some transsexuals the need for treatment that results in gender reassignment may be of paramount importance. However, not all transsexuals will choose to change the physical aspects of their body image. For those patients who have or are in the process of gender reassignment, the transformation will be as much cognitive, emotional and social as physical. The clinical decision about gender reassignment surgery is usually arrived at in two phases. In the first phase – a period of psychodiagnostic assessment – information is gathered on individuals' general psychosexual development, their sexual behaviour and sexual orientation, the subject of their cross-dressing and their body image. An individual's intellectual and emotional coping mechanisms will be appraised and assessment made to detect psychopathology (Cohen-Kettenis and Gooren, 1999). The requirements of the second phase are to live openly and permanently in the role of the desired sex for two years, this is sometimes referred to as the 'real-life test' (Wilson, 2000). During this time, regular contact with a knowledgeable psychiatrist or psychologist is required. Some treatment centres will require patients to do this successfully for a period of time before commencing hormone treatment, whereas others prescribe hormone treatment as soon as cross-gender living has started. The first effects of hormone treatment become apparent after a few months, but it may take many years before the changes are complete (Asscheman and Gooren, 1992). Some clinicians will also require their patients to undertake a certain number of psychotherapy sessions prior to medical treatment. This can be problematic not least because some transsexuals fear, sometimes correctly, that they will be denied gender reassignment treatment if they are honest about their problems during psychotherapy. Cohen-Kettenis and Gooren (1999) state that the idea behind these requirements is that the individual should have the opportunity to appreciate in fantasy or *in vivo* the consequences of gender role change, as well as exploring any doubts about sex reassignment surgery or unresolved personal issues before any irreversible physical changes occur. Critics of such exacting pre-treatment requirements, however, suggest that these lengthen the process of gender reassignment unnecessarily as well as making it more expensive.

When an individual is deemed to have effected a satisfactory social role change during the 'real life test', he or she is referred for surgery. The surgery for male-to-female transsexuals involves vaginoplasty and sometimes breast enlargement. For female-to-male transsexuals surgery includes breast reduction and hysterectomy. Some patients may have phalloplasty (still a relatively experimental procedure), whereas other will elect to have a neoscrotum with testicular prosthesis and surgery to transform the hypertrophic clitoris into a microphallus. Bland (1998) notes that in the UK under NHS procedures once surgery is completed, the process of treatment and care is considered finished. If further help is required, an individual has to seek this as a new patient. According to Bland (1998), however, many post-operative transsexuals simply wish to disappear quietly back into the community.

As can be seen from the above, the process of seeking and obtaining gender reassignment surgery is a protracted and often turbulent one. Transsexuals are required to subject their most intimate feelings, thoughts and behaviours to the scrutiny of clinicians – some of whom will have the authority to sanction or deny surgery – whilst adapting to a huge transformation of their social self as well as the physical and emotional changes effected by hormone treatment. The psychosexual anxiety and distress felt by patients at this time in their lives may be particularly great as they face the prospect of 'coming out' to family, friends and colleagues – often at the onset of their 'real-life' test, dealing with loss and adjusting to change and uncertainty during the period of reassignment. For patients who have completed the process of physical change associated with gender reassignment, it should be remembered that change does not cease with the cessation of surgery. Zandvliet (2000), commenting on some of his clients who have been through medically successful treatment, observes that:

> At the end of the physical treatment they felt at a loss about almost everything: their emotions, their past, their relationships and their sexuality. Transformation is a mental, social and cultural process: from my viewpoint a process of migration. (Zanvliet, 2000, p. 186)

Furthermore, transsexuals, whether or not they have undergone gender reassignment, often have to endure considerable discrimination, isolation and rejection (Turner, 1999; Wilson, 2000). Some individuals do not seek complete surgical reassignment, preferring to try to integrate masculine and feminine aspects of the self and thus seek only partial medical treatment, either hormone treatment or only some forms of surgery. Those not seeking complete gender reassignment are sometimes called 'transgenderists'. The transgenderist challenges the rigid concept of just two sexes, which is the premise for medical treatment. Consequently, it may be often more difficult for a transgenderist to obtain medical support for treatment. For patients who are experiencing distress related to issues concerning their own or their partner's gender identity, the support of the Gender Trust (*see* Appendix I) may be helpful.

Key points of Chapter 10

- Individuals are only likely to present for help with sexual variations or issues relating to gender identity if these are causing anxiety or distress or are adversely affecting their relationship with others.
- Although the management of such problems is a specialist matter, the recognition and acknowledgement of the distress or anxiety felt by patients is something all practitioners can offer.
- Patients require care that respects their individuality and recognizes them as a whole person and not just a diagnostic category.
- Some of the anxieties and fears evoked in practitioners by sexual difference may correspond to some of the feelings experienced by patients and their partners.
- Not all transsexuals will elect to undergo gender reassignment, those that do are faced with vast numbers of changes – emotional, cognitive and social as well as those that are physical – before, during and after the gender reassignment process.
- Although gender reassignment may substantially alleviate the suffering of many people with gender dysphoria, it is no panacea.

Key reading

Cohen-Kettenis, P.T., Gooren, L.J.G. (1999) Transsexualism: a review of etiology, diagnosis and treatment. *Journal of Psychosomatic Research* **46**; 4: 315–333.
Headon, C.F. (1998) A counsellor's work with clients presenting with paraphilias. In: Freeman, H., Pullen, I., Stein, G., Wilkinson, G. (eds). *Seminars in Psychosexual Disorders*. London: Gaskell.

APPENDIX I

Useful addresses

Association to Aid the Sexual and Personal Relationships of People with a Disability (SPOD)
286 Camden Road
London N7 0BJ
Telephone: 020 7607 8851 (Helpline: Tuesday and Thursday 11 am to 2 pm)

Association of Psychosexual Nursing
PO Box 2762
London W1A 5HQ

Beaumont Trust
BM Charity
London WC1N 3XX
(Helpline for transsexuals, transvestites and their partners)
Telephone: 07000 287878 (Tuesday and Thursday 7 pm to 11 pm)

British Association for Sexual and Relationship Therapy
PO Box 13686
London SW20 9ZH
Website: www.basrt.org.uk

British Pregnancy Advisory Service (BPAS)
Austy Manor
Wootton Wawen, Solihull
West Midlands B95 6BX
Telephone: 08457 304030
Website: www.bpas.org

CancerBACUP
3 Bath Place
Rivington Street
London EC2A 3JR
Telephone: 0808 800 1234
Website: www.cancerbacup.org.uk

Child: Infertility Education Counselling
Charter House
43 St Leonards Road
Bexhill on Sea
East Sussex TN40 1JA
Website: www.child.org.uk

Gender Trust
PO Box 3192
Brighton BN1 3WR
Telephone: 07000 790347

Impotence Association
PO Box 10296
London SW17 9WH
Helpline: 020 8767 7791 (Monday to Friday 9 am to 5 pm)
Website: www.impotence.org.uk

Institute of Psychosexual Medicine
12 Chandos Street
Cavendish Square
London W1G 9DR
Telephone: 020 7580 0631
Website: www.ipm.org.uk

Issue (National Fertility Association)
114 Lichfield Street
Walsall
West Midlands WS1 1SZ
Telephone: 01922 722888
Website: www.issue.co.uk

London Lesbian and Gay Switchboard
PO Box 7324
London N1 9QS
Telephone: 020 7837 7324

Relate
Relate Central Office
Herbert Gray College
Little Church Street
Rugby
Warwickshire CV21 3AP
Telephone: 01788 573241
Helpline: 01372 464100
Website: www.relate.org.uk

Society of Health Advisors in Sexually Transmitted Diseases (SHASTD)
MSF Centre
33–37 Moreland Street
London EC1V 8BB
Website: www.shastd.org.uk

Stillbirth and Neonatal Death Society (SANDS)
28 Portland Place
London W1N 4DE
Telephone: 020 7436 5881
Website: www.uk-sands.org

The Miscarriage Association
c/o Clayton Hospital
Northgate
Wakefield
West Yorkshire WF1 3JS
Helpline: 01924 200799 (Monday to Friday 9 am to 4 pm)
Scottish helpline: 0131 334 8883 (answerphone with names of local contacts)

APPENDIX II

Bibliography for further reading

Bancroft, J. (1989) *Human Sexuality and Its Problems* (second edition). Edinburgh: Churchill Livingstone.

Borwell, B. (ed.) (1997) *Developing Sexual Helping Skills: A Guide for Nurses*. Maidenhead: Medical Projects International.

Daines, B., Perrett, A. (2000) *Psychodynamic Approaches to Sexual Problems*. Buckingham: Open University Press.

Freeman, H., Pullen, I., Stein, G., Wilkinson, G. (eds) (1998) *Seminars in Psychosexual Disorders*. London: Gaskell.

Hawton, K. (1985) *Sex Therapy: A Practical Guide*. Oxford: Oxford University Press.

Heath, H., White, I. (eds) (2001) *The Challenge of Sexuality in Health Care*. Oxford: Blackwell Science.

Miller, D., Green, J. (eds) (2002) *The Psychology of Sexual Health*. Oxford: Blackwell Science.

Montford, H., Skrine, R. (eds) (1993) *Contraceptive Care: Meeting Individual Needs*. London: Chapman & Hall.

Nichols, K.A. (1993) *Psychological Care in Physical Illness* (second edition). London: Chapman & Hall.

Nye, R. (ed.) (1999) *Sexuality*. Oxford: Oxford University Press.

Parkes, C.M., Markus, A. (eds) (1998) *Coping with Loss*. London: BMJ Books.

Petrak, J., Hedge, B. (eds) (2002) *The Trauma of Sexual Assault*. Chichester: John Wiley & Sons Ltd.

Savage, J. (1987) *Nurses, Gender and Sexuality*. London: Heinemann Nursing.

Skrine, R.L. (ed.) (1989) *Introduction to Psychosexual Medicine*. Carlisle: Montana Press.

Skrine, R., Montford, H. (eds) (2001) *Psychosexual Medicine: An Introduction* (second edition). London: Arnold.

Tiefer, L. (1995) *Sex Is Not A Natural Act*. Oxford: Westview Press.

Ussher, J.M., Baker, C.D. (eds) (1993) *Psychological Perspectives on Sexual Problems*. London: Routledge.

Webb, C. (1985) *Sexuality Nursing and Health*. Chichester: John Wiley & Sons.

Wells, D. (ed.) (2000) *Caring for Sexuality in Health and Illness*. Edinburgh: Churchill Livingstone.

References

Adler, M.W. (1998) Sexual health. *British Medical Journal* **317**, 1479.

Albarran, J.W., Salmon, D. (2000) Lesbian, gay and bisexual experiences within critical care nursing 1988–1998: a survey of the literature. *International Journal of Nursing Studies* **37**, 445–455.

Altschuler, J. (1997) *Working with Chronic Illness*. London: Macmillan.

APA (1995) *Diagnostic and Statistical Manual of Mental Disorder* (fourth edition), International Version. Washington DC: American Psychiatric Association.

Andersen, B.L. (1990) How cancer affects sexual functioning. *Oncology* **4**, 6, 81–88.

Annon, J.S. (1976) The P-LI-SS-IT model: a proposed conceptual scheme for the behavioural treatment of sexual problems. *Journal of Sex Education and Therapy* **2**, 1–15.

Asscheman, H., Gooren, L.J.G. (1992) Hormone treatment in transsexuals. *Journal of Psychology and Human Sexuality* **5**, 39–54.

Aston, G. (2001) Sexuality during and after pregnancy. In: Andrews, G. (ed.) *Women's Sexual Health* (second edition). London: Baillière Tindall.

Baker, C.D., de Silva, P. (1988) The relationship between male sexual dysfunction and belief in Zilbergeld's myths: an empirical investigation. *Sexual and Marital Therapy* **3**, 2, 229–238.

Bancroft, J. (1989) *Human Sexuality and Its Problems* (second edition). Edinburgh: Churchill Livingstone.

Barclay, L.M., McDonald, P., O'Loughlin, J.A. (1994) Sexuality and pregnancy an interview study. *Australian and New Zealand Journal of Obstetrics and Gynaecology* **34**, 1–7.

Barlow, D.H. (1986) Causes of sexual dysfunction: the role of anxiety and cognitive interference. *Journal of Consulting and Clinical Psychology* **54**, 2, 140–148.

Barnes, E., Griffiths, P., Ord, J., Wells, D. (eds) (1998) *Face to Face with Distress: The Professional Use of Self in Psychosocial Care*. Oxford: Butterworth–Heinemann.

Barrett, G., Pendry, E., Peacock, J., Victor, C., Thakar, R., Manyonda, I. (2000) Women's sexual health after childbirth. *BJOG: An International Journal of Obstetrics and Gynaecology* **107**, 2, 186–195.

Bartellas, E., Crane, J.M.G., Daley, M., Bennett, K.A., Hutchens, D. (2000) Sexuality and sexual activity in pregnancy. *BJOG: An International Journal of Obstetrics and Gynaecology* **107**, 964–968.

Bartlett, A., King, M., Phillips, P. (2001) Straight taking: an investigation of the attitudes and practice of psychoanalysts and psychotherapists in relation to gays and lesbians. *British Journal of Psychiatry* **179**, 545–549.

Barton, S., Jewitt, C. (1995) Talking about about sex. In: Curtis, H., Hoolaghan, T., Jewitt, C. (eds) *Sexual Health Promotion in General Practice*. Abingdon: Radcliffe Medical.

Basson, R. (2001) Human sex-response cycles. *Journal of Sex and Marital Therapy* **27**, 33–43.

Basson, R., Berman, J., Burnett, A., Dergotis, L., Ferguson, D., Fourcoy, J. et al. (2000) Report of the International Consensus Development Conference on Female Sexual Dysfunction: Definitions and Classifications. *Journal of Urology* **163,** 888–893.

Beauchamp, T.L., Childress, J.F. (1989) *Principles of Biomedical Ethics* (third edition). New York: Oxford University Press.

Bell, R. (1999) Homosexual men and women. ABC of sexual health. *British Medical Journal* **318**, 452–455

Berman, J., Berman, L. (2001) *For Women Only*. London: Virago Press.

Berry, M. (1997) Coming to terms with sexual abuse. *British Journal of Sexual Medicine* **24**, 3, 10–13.

Berry, M. (1999) Grief and psychosexual disturbance following the death of a young baby: some issues for practitioners. *Sexual and Marital Therapy* **14**, 1, 27–42.

Bhui, K. (1998) Psychosexual care in a multi-ethnic society. *Journal of the Royal Society of Medicine* **91**, 141–143.

Bignell, C.J. (1999) Chaperones for genital examination. *British Medical Journal* **319**, 137–138.

Bland, J. (1998) Transgenderism and the psychiatrist. In: Freeman, H., Pullen, I., Stein, G., Wilkinson, G. (eds) *Seminars in Psychosexual Disorders*. London: Gaskell.

Boag, F., Barton, S.E. (1993) Psychosexual aspects of sexually transmitted diseases. *Medicine International* **21**, 3, 107–108.

Bor, R., Watts, M. (1993) Talking to patients about sexual matters. *British Journal of Nursing* **2**, 13, 657–661.

Bor, R., Scher, I. (1995) A family-systems approach to infertility counselling. In: Jennings, S.E. (ed.) *Infertility Counselling*. Oxford: Blackwell Science.

Bor, R., Miller, R., Latz, M., Salt, H. (1998) *Counselling in Health Care Settings*. London: Cassell.

Borwell, B. (ed.) (1997) *Developing Sexual Helping Skills: A Guide for Nurses*. Maidenhead: Medical Projects International.

Botell, J. (2001) Training lectures in psychosexual medicine: skills of psychosexual medicine. *Institute of Psychosexual Medicine Journal* **26**, February, 24–29.

Brandt, A.M., Jones, D.S. (1999) Historical perspectives on sexually transmitted diseases: challenges for prevention and control. In: Holmes, K.K. et al. (eds) *Sexually Transmitted Diseases* (third edition). New York: McGraw-Hill.

Briant, S. (1997) Too close for comfort. *Nursing Times* **93**, 6, 22–24.

Brien, J., Fairbairn, I. (1996) *Pregnancy and Abortion Counselling*. London: Routledge.

Bulik, C.M., Prescott, C.A., Kendler, K.S. (2001) Features of childhood sexual abuse and the development of psychiatric and substance use disorders. *British Journal of Psychiatry* **179**, 444–449.

Burnard, P. (2000) Talking about sexuality: a challenge for community nurses. *Journal of Community Nursing* **14**, 3, 13–16.

Burnett, A., Peel, M (2001) The health of survivors or torture and organized violence. *British Medical Journal* **322**, 606–609.

Butcher, J. (1999) Female sexual problems 1: Loss of desire – what about fun? ABC of sexual health. *British Medical Journal* **318**, 41–43.

Butler, C., Joyce, V. (1998) *Counselling Couples in Relationships*. Chichester: John Wiley & Sons Ltd.

Caruso, S., Intelisano, G., Lupo, L., Agnello, C. (2001) Premenopausal women affected by sexual arousal disorder treated with sidenafil: a double-blind, cross-over, placebo-controlled study. *British Journal of Obstetrics and Gynaecology* **108**, 623–628.

Catalan, J. (ed.) (1999) *Mental Health and HIV Infection: Psychological and Psychiatric Aspects.* London: UCL Press.

Catalan, J., Thornton, S. (1999) Mental health. In: Gazzard, B. (ed.) *Chelsea & Westminster Hospital AIDS Care Handbook.* London: Mediscript Ltd Medical Publishers.

Catalan, J., Hawton, K, Day, A. (1990) Couples referred to a sexual dysfunction clinic: psychological and physical morbidity. *British Journal of Psychiatry* **156**, 61–67.

Catalan, J., Hawton, K., Day, A. (1991) Individuals presenting without partners at a sexual dysfunction clinic: psychological and physical morbidity and treatment offered. *Sexual and Marital Therapy* **6**, 15–23.

Catalan, J., Bradley, M., Gallwey, J., Hawton, K. (1981) Sexual dysfunction and psychiatric morbidity in patients attending a clinic for sexually transmitted diseases. *British Journal of Psychiatry* **138**, 292–296.

Catalan, J., Burgess, A., Klimes, I. (1995) *Psychological Medicine of HIV Infection.* Oxford: Oxford University Press.

Caufield, H., Platzer, H. (1998) Next of kin. *Nursing Standard* **13**, 7, 47–49.

Cavicchia, S., Whitehead, B. (1995) Professional development, counselling approaches to health promotion and motivational skills. In: Curtis, H., Hoolaghan, T., Jewitt, C. (eds) *Sexual Health Promotion in General Practice.* Oxford: Radcliffe Medical Press.

Champion, A. (1996) Male cancer and sexual function. *Sexual and Marital Therapy* **11**, 3, 227–244.

Chippendale, S., French, L. (2001) HIV counselling and the psychosocial management of patients with HIV or AIDS. ABC of AIDS. *British Medical Journal* **322**, (7301), 1533–1535.

Christopher, E. (1993) Unconscious factors in contraceptive care: understanding ambivalence and poor motivation. In: Montford, H., Skrine, R. (eds) *Contraceptive Care: Meeting Individual Needs.* London: Chapman & Hall.

Christopher, E. (1996) *Counselling People with Psycho-Sexual Problems.* Guidebooks for Counsellors, Rugby: British Association for Counselling.

Clifford, D. (1998a) Psychosexual nursing seminars. In: Barnes, E., Griffiths, P., Ord, J., Wells, D. (eds) *Face to Face with Distress: The Professional Use of the Self in Psychosocial Care.* Oxford: Butterworth–Heinemann.

Clifford, D. (1998b) Psychosexual awareness in everyday nursing. *Nursing Standard* **12**, 39, 42–45.

Clifford, D. (2000a) Section 1 Developing psychosexual awareness (chapters 1–6). In: Wells, D. (ed.) *Caring for Sexuality in Health and Illness.* Edinburgh: Churchill Livingstone.

Clifford, D. (2000b) The Hidden Work of Nursing. Caring for Sexuality in Health and Illness. Papers given at the study day on 18 November, 2000 organized by the Association of Psychosexual Nursing with the Liverpool Women's Hospital. London: Association of Psychosexual Nursing.

Cohen-Kettinis, P.T., Gooren, L.R.G. (1999) Transsexualism: a review of etiology, diagnosis and treatment. *Journal of Psychosomatic Research* **46**, 4, 315–333.

Cole, J. (1997) Psychosexual therapy and Relate. *British Journal of Sexual Medicine* **24**, 1, 18–21.

Cole, S.W., Kemeny, M.E., Taylor, S.E., Visscher, B.R. (1996) Elevated physical health risk among gay men who conceal their homosexual identity. *Health Psychology* **15**, 4, 243–251.

Coleman, E., Hoon, P., Hoon, H. (1983) Arousability and sexual satisfaction in lesbian and heterosexual women. *Journal of Sex Research* **19**, 58–73.

Coleman, R., Etchegoyen, A. (1992) The psychodynamics of the STD clinic: secrecy, splitting and isolation. *British Journal of Medical Psychology* **65**, 319–326.

Cooper, G.F. (1988) The psychological methods of sex therapy. In: Cole, M., Dryden, W. (eds) *Sex Therapy in Britain*. Buckingham: Open University Press.

Coxell, A., King, M., Mezey, G., Gordon, D. (1999) Lifetime prevalence, characteristics, and associated problems of non-consensual sex in men: cross sectional survey. *British Medical Journal* **318**, 846–850.

Coxon, A.P.M. (1996) *Between the Sheets: Sexual Diaries and Gay Men's Sex in the Era of AIDS*. London: Cassell.

Creighton, S. (2001) Surgery for intersex. *Journal of the Royal Society of Medicine* **94**, 218–220.

Creighton, S., Minto, C. (2001) Managing intersex. *British Medical Journal* **323**, 1264–1265.

Crowe, M. (1998) Sexual therapy and the couple. In: Freeman, H., Pullen, I., Stein, G., Wilkinson, G. (eds) *Seminars in Psychosexual Disorders*. London: Gaskell.

Crowe, M., Ridley, J. (2000) *Therapy with Couples*. Oxford: Blackwell Science.

Crowley, T. (1997) Psychosexual medicine in a genitourinary medicine clinic. *Institute of Psychosexual Medicine Journal* **16**, September, 5–9.

Crowley, T. (2001a) Sexual problems when the partner is of the same gender. *Institute of Psychosexual Medicine Journal* **26**, February, 12–17.

Crowley, T. (2001b) The genito-urinary clinic. In: Skrine, R., Montford, H. (eds) *Psychosexual Medicine: An Introduction*. London: Arnold.

Crowther, M.E., Corney, R.H., Shepherd, J.H. (1994) Psychosexual implications of gynaecological cancer. *British Medical Journal* **308**, 869–870.

Cull, A., Cowie, V.J., Farquharson, D.I.M., Livingstone, J.R.B., Smart, G.E., Elton, R.A. (1993) Early stage cervical cancer: psychosocial and sexual outcomes of treatment. *British Journal of Cancer* **68**, 1216–1220.

Cybulska, B., Forster, G. (2001) Sexual assault: examination of the victim. *Medicine* **29**, 7, 32–36.

Daines, B., Perrett, A. (2000) *Psychodynamic Approaches to Sexual Problems*. Buckingham: Open University Press.

D'Ardenne, P. (1988) Sexual dysfunction in a transcultural setting. In: Cole, M., Dryden, W. (eds) *Sex Therapy in Britain*. Buckingham: Open University Press.

Davies, D. (1996a) Homophobia and heterosexism. In: Davies, D., Neal, C. (eds) *Pink Therapy: A Guide for Counsellors and Therapists Working with Lesbian, Gay and Bisexual Clients*. Buckingham: Open University Press.

Davies, D. (1996b) Working with people coming out. In: Davies, D., Neal, C. (eds) *Pink Therapy: A Guide for Counsellors and Therapists Working with Lesbian, Gay and Bisexual Clients*. Buckingham: Open University Press.

Davies, D. (1996c) Working with young people. In: Davies, D., Neal, C. (eds) *Pink Therapy: A Guide for Counsellors and Therapists Working with Lesbian, Gay and Bisexual Clients*. Buckingham: Open University Press.

Davis, M. (2001) Painful intercourse. In: Skrine, R., Montford, H. (eds) *Psychosexual Medicine* (second edition). London: Arnold.

Dean, J. (1998) Examination of patients with sexual problems. ABC of sexual health. *British Medical Journal* **317**, 1641–1643.

De Raeve, L. (1998) Knowing patients: how much and how well? In: Barnes, E., Griffiths, P., Ord, J., Wells, D. (eds) *Face to Face with Distress: The Professional Use of Self in Psychosocial Care*. Oxford: Butterworth–Heineman.

De Silva, W.P. (1999) Sexual variations. ABC of sexual health. *British Medical Journal* **318**, 654–656.

Denman, F. (1993) Prejudice and homosexuality. *British Journal of Psychotherapy* **9**, 346–358.

Denman, M. (1995) Psychosexual problems at the menopause. *British Journal of Sexual Medicine* March/April, 8–9.

Department of Health (2001a) *The National Strategy for Sexual Health and HIV*. Consultation Document, London: Department of Health.

Department of Health (2001b) *Treatment Choice in Psychological Therapies and Counselling: Evidence Based Clinical Practice Guideline*. London: Department of Health.

Derman, R.J. (1986) Counselling the herpes genitalis patient. *Journal of Reproductive Medicine* **31**, 439–445.

Dixon, M., Booth, N., Powell, R. (2000) Sex and relationships following childbirth: a first report from general practice of 131 couples. *British Journal of General Practice* **50**, 223–224.

Doyle, G. (1998) Child abuse. In: Freeman, H., Pullen, I., Stein, G., Wilkinson, G. (eds) *Seminars in Psychosexual Disorders*. London: Gaskell.

Drob, S., Loeman, M., Lifschutz, H. (1985) Genital herpes: the psychological consequences. *British Journal of Medical Psychology* **58**, 307–315.

Dryden, W. (1985) Sex therapy: education or healing? An interview with John Bancroft. In: Dryden, W. *Therapist's Dilemmas*. London: Sage Publications.

Dudley, W. (1995) The psychological impact of warts on patients' lives. *Professional Nurse* **11**, 2, 99–100.

Duncan, B., Hart, G. (1999) Sexuality and health: the hidden costs of screening for Chlamydia trachomatis. *British Medical Journal* **318**, 931–933.

Duncan, B., Hart, G., Scoular, A., Bigrigg, A. (2001) Qualitative analysis of psychosocial impact of diagnosis of Chlamydia trachomatis: implications for screening. *British Medical Journal* **322**, 195–199.

Dunn, K.M., Croft, P.R., Hackett, G.I. (1998) Sexual problems: a study of the prevalence and need for health care in the general population. *Family Practice* **15**, 6, 519–524.

Egan, G. (1990) *The Skilled Helper: A Systematic Approach to Effective Helping* (fourth edition). Pacific Grove, CA: Brooks Cole Publishing Company.

Ellis, A., Dryden, W. (1999) *The Practice of Rational Emotive Behavioural Therapy* (second edition). London: Free Association Books.

ENB (1994) *Caring for People with Sexually Transmitted Diseases, including HIV Disease*. Open Learning Pack. London: English National Board for Nursing, Midwifery and Health Visiting.

Fabricius, J. (1991) Running on the spot or can nursing really change? *Psychoanalytic Psychotherapy* **5**, 2, 97–108.

Finkelhor, D., Browne, A. (1985) The traumatic impact of child sexual abuse: a conceptualization. *American Journal of Orthopsychiatry* **55**, 4, 530–541.

Finnis, S.J., Robbins, I. (1994) Sexual harassment of nurses: an occupational hazard? *Journal of Clinical Nursing* **3**, 87–95.

Firn, S. (1996) Marrying mind and matter. In: Faugier, J., Hicken, I. (eds) *AIDS and HIV: The Nursing Response*. London: Chapman & Hall.

Freeman, H., Pullen, I., Stein, G., Wilkinson, G. (eds) *Seminars in Psychosexual Disorders*. London: Gaskell.

Friedman, D. (1988) Assessing the basis of sexual dysfunction: diagnostic procedures. In Cole, M., Dryden, W. (eds) *Sex Therapy in Britain*. Buckingham: Open University Press.

Frost, D.P. (1985) Recognition of hypochondriasis in a clinic for sexually transmitted disease. *Genitourinary Medicine* **61**, 133–137.

Gabbott, M., Jones, A., O'Brien, D, Roberts, M. (1999) Can a couple be a patient? *Institute of Psychosexual Medicine Journal* **25**, January, 3–7.

Gamlin, R. (1999) Sexuality: a challenge for nursing practice. *Nursing Times* **95**, 7, 48–50.

George, H (1993) Sex, love and relationships: issues and problems for gay men in the AIDS era. In: Ussher, J.M., Baker, C.D. (eds) *Psychological Perspectives on Sexual Problems*. London: Routledge.

George, H. (1994) Sexual and relationship problems among people affected by AIDS: three case studies. In: Bor, R., Elford, J. (eds) *The Family and HIV*. London: Cassell.

Gibson, H.B. (1992) *The Emotional and Sexual Lives of Older People: A Manual for Professionals*. London: Chapman & Hall.

Gill, M. (2001) Interaction of physical and psychological factors. In: Skrine, R., Montford, H. (eds) *Psychosexual Medicine: An Introduction* (second edition). London: Arnold.

Gilmore, N., Somerville, M.A. (1994) Stigmatization, scapegoating and discrimination in sexually transmitted diseases: overcoming 'them' and 'us'. *Social Science and Medicine* **39**, 9, 1339–1358.

Glass, C., Soni, B. (1999) Sexual problems of disabled patients. ABC of sexual health. *British Medical Journal* **318**, 518–521.

Glover, J. (1985) *Human Sexuality in Nursing Care*. Beckenham: Croom Helm Ltd.

Glover, L., Abel, P.D., Gannon, K. (1998) Male subfertility: is pregnancy the only issue? *British Medical Journal* **316**, 1405–1406.

Golding, J. (1997) *Without Prejudice: MIND Lesbian, Gay and Bisexual Mental Health Awareness Research*. London: MIND Publications.

Goldmeier, D. (2001) Female low sexual desire and sexually transmitted infections. *Sexually Transmitted Infections* **77**, 293–294.

Goldmeier, D., Keane, F.E.A., Carter, P., Hessman, A., Harris, J.R.W., Renton, A. (1997) Prevalence of sexual dysfunction in heterosexual patients attending a central London genitourinary medicine clinic. *International Journal of STD and AIDS* **8**, 303–306.

Golombok, S., Fivush, R. (1998) Gender development. In: Freeman, H., Pullen, I., Stein, G., Wilkinson, G. (eds) *Seminars in Psychosexual Disorders*. London: Gaskell.

Gonsiorek, J.C. (1982) Results of psychological testing of homosexual populations. *American Behavioral Scientist* **25**, 385–396.

Gordon, P. (1988) Sex therapy with gay men. In: Cole, M., Dryden, W. (eds) *Sex Therapy in Britain*. Buckingham: Open University Press.

Gould, D.C., Petty, R., Jacobs, H.S. (2000) For and against: the male menopause – does it exist? *British Medical Journal* **320**, 858–861.

Green, C. (1999) Clause 9: Honouring professional contact. In: Heywood Jones, I. (ed.) *UKCC Code of Professional Conduct – A Critical Guide*. London: Nursing Times Books.

Green, J., Kentish, J. (1986) The worried well. In: Green, J., McCreaner, A. (eds) *Counselling in HIV Infection and AIDS* (second edition). Oxford: Blackwell Science.

Gregoire, A. (1999a) Male sexual problems. ABC of sexual health. *British Medical Journal* **318**, 518–521.

Gregoire, A. (1999b) Assessing and managing male sexual problems. ABC of sexual health. *British Medical Journal* **318**, 315–317.

Gregory, P. (1999) Psychosexual therapy. *Nursing Standard* **13**, 48, 37–40.

Grigg, E. (1999) Sexuality and older people. *Elderly Care* **11**, 7, 12–15.

Grubin, D. (1999) Therapist or public protector? Ethical responses to anti-social sexual behaviour. *Sexual and Marital Therapy* **14**, 3, 277–288.

Guthrie, C. (1999) Nurses' perceptions of sexuality relating to patient care. *Journal of Clinical Nursing* **8**, 313–321.

Haldemann, D. (1991) Sexual orientation conversion therapy for gay men and lesbians: a scientific examination. In: Gonsiorek, J., Weinrich, J. (eds) *Homosexuality: Research Implications for Public Policy*. Newbridge Park, CA: Sage.

Hancock, K.A. (1995) Psychotherapy with lesbians and gay men. In: d'Augelli, A.R., Patterson, C.J. (eds) *Lesbian, Gay and Bisexual Identities Over the Lifespan: Psychological Perspectives*. Oxford: Oxford University Press.

Hardman, A., Jones, J., Scott, D.A., Stevens, J. (1998) Unwanted sexual experiences reported by nursing students: implications for nurse education and training. *Journal of Advanced Nursing* **28**, 5, 1158–1167.

Hart, G., Welling, K. (2002) Sexual behaviour and its medicalisation: in sickness and in health. *British Medical Journal* **324**, 896–900.

Hartmann, J.T., Albrecht, C., Schmoll, H-J., Kuczyk, M.A., Kollmannsberger, C., Bokemeyer, C. (1999) Long-term effects on sexual function and fertility after treatment of testicular cancer. *British Journal of Cancer* **80**, 5/6, 801–807.

Hawton, K. (1985) *Sex Therapy: A Practical Guide*. Oxford: Oxford University Press.

Hawton, K. (1995) Treatment of sexual dysfunction by sex therapy and other approaches. *British Journal of Psychiatry* **167**, 307–314.

Hayter, M. (1996) Is non-judgemental care possible in the context of nurses' attitudes to patients' sexuality. *Journal of Advanced Nursing* **24**, 662–666.

Hayter, M. (1999) Prophylaxis to combat HIV infection after sexual exposure. *Nursing Times* **95**, 23, 44–45.

Headon, C.F. (1998) A counsellor's work with clients presenting with paraphilias. In: Freeman, H., Pullen, I., Stein, G., Wilkinson, G. (eds) *Seminars in Psychosexual Disorders*. London: Gaskell.

Heath, H. (2001) Sexuality and later life. In: Heath, H., White, I. (eds) *The Challenge of Sexuality for Health Care*. Oxford: Blackwell Science.

Heath, H., White, I. (eds) (2001) *The Challenge of Sexuality for Health Care*. Oxford: Blackwell Science.

Hedge, B. (1999) The impact of HIV infection on partners and relatives. In: Catalan, J. (ed.) *Mental Health and HIV Infection: Psychological and Psychiatric Aspects*. London: UCL Press.

Hedge, B. (2002) Coping with the physical impact of sexual assault. In: Petrak, J., Hedge, B. (eds) *The Trauma of Sexual Assault*. Chichester: John Wiley and Sons Ltd.

Hennebry, G. (1998) Being heard. *Nursing Times* **94**, 17, 26–28.

Hicken, I. (1994) *Sexual Health Education and Training: Guidelines for Good Practice and the Teaching of Nurses, Midwives and Health Visitors*. London: English National Board for Nursing, Midwifery and Health Visiting.

Hickerton, M. (2001) Women with special needs and concerns. In: Andrews, G. (ed.) *Women's Sexual Health* (second edition). London: Baillière Tindall; pp 109–133.

Hitchings, P. (1997) Counselling and sexual orientation. In: Palmer, S., McMahon, G. (eds) *Handbook of Counselling* (second edition). London: Routledge.

Hobbs, K., Bramwell, R., May, K. (1999) Sexuality, sexual behaviour and pregnancy. *Sexual and Marital Therapy* **14**, 4, 371–383.

Holgate, H.S., Longman, C. (1998) Some peoples' psychological experiences of attending a sexual health clinic and having a sexually transmitted infection. *Journal of the Royal Society of Health* **118**, 2, 94–96.

Huish, M., Kumar, D., Stones, C. (1998) Stoma surgery and sexual problems in ostomates. *Sexual and Marital Therapy* **13**, 3, 311–328.

Hutchinson, H. (2001) The psychosexual medicine clinic. In: Skrine, R., Montford, H. (eds) *Psychosexual Medicine: An Introduction* (second edition). London: Arnold.

Ikkos, G., Fitzpatrick, R., Frost, D., Nazeer, S. (1997) Psychological disturbance and illness behaviour in a clinic for sexually transmitted diseases. *British Journal of Medical Psychology* **60**, 121–126.

IPM (1995) *Prospectus*. London: Institute of Psychosexual Medicine.

Irving, G., Miller, D., Robinson, A., Reynolds, S., Copas, A.J. (1998) Psychological factors associated with recurrent vaginal candidiasis: a preliminary study. *Sexually Transmitted Infections* **74**, 334–338.

Jehu, D. (1991) Clinical work with adults who were sexually abused as children. In: Hollin, C.R., Howelles, K. (eds) *Clinical Approaches to Sex Offenders and Their Victims*. Chichester: Wiley.

Jenkins, P. (1999) Client or patient? Contrasts between medical and counselling models of confidentiality. *Counselling Psychology Quarterly* **12**, 2, 169–181.

Johnson, A.M., Wadsworth, J., Wellings, K., Field, J. (1996) Who goes to sexually transmitted disease clinics? Results from a national population survey. *Genitourinary Medicine* **72**, 197–202.

Johnson, M., Webb, C. (1995) Rediscovering the unpopular patient: the concept of social judgement. *Journal of Advanced Nursing* **21**, 466–475.

Jones, C., Nugent, P. (2001) The problem of erectile dysfunction following myocardial infarction. *Professional Nurse* **17**, 3, 161–164.

Kaplan, H.S. (1974) *The New Sex Therapy*. New York: Brunner/Mazel.

Kaplan, H.S. (1977) Hypoactive sexual desire. *Journal of Sex and Marital Therapy* **3**, 3–9.

Kaplan, H.S. (1979) *Disorders of Sexual Desire*. London: Baillière Tindall.

Kautz, D.D., Dickey, C.A., Stevens, M.N. (1990) Using research to identify why nurses do not meet established sexuality nursing care standards. *Journal of Nursing Quality Assurance* **4**, 3, 69–78.

Keane, F.E.A., Carter, P, Goldmeier, D., Harris, J.R.W. (1997) The provision of psychosexual services by genitourinary medicine physicians in the United Kingdom. *International Journal of STD and AIDS* **8**, 402–404.

Kell, P. (2001) The provision of sexual dysfunction services by genitourinary medicine physicians in the UK, 1999. *International Journal of STD and AIDS* **12**, 395–397.

Kelly, D. (2001) Sexuality and people with acute illness. In: Heath, H., White, I. (eds) *The Challenge of Sexuality in Health Care*. Oxford: Blackwell Science.

Kennerley, H. (2002) Managing the sequelae of childhood sexual abuse in adults. In: Miller, D., Green, J. (eds) *The Psychology of Sexual Health*. Oxford: Blackwell Science.

King, E. (1998) *Post-exposure Prophylaxis (PEP) Against HIV Infection Following Sexual and Injection Drug Use Exposure*. NHPIS Briefing 1. National HIV Prevention Information Service, Health Education Authority, London.

Kitzinger, J.V. (1992) Counteracting, not reenacting, the violation of women's bodies: the challenge for perinatal caregivers. *Birth* **19**, 219.

Lab, D. (2000) Sexual health abused. In: Wilson, H., McAndrew, S. (eds) *Sexual Health*. London: Baillière Tindall.

Lacey, H. (1999) National Guidelines on the Management of Adult Victims of Sexual Assault. Clinical Effectiveness Group (Association of Genitourinary Medicine and the Medical Society for the Study of Venereal Diseases). *Sexually Transmitted Infections* **75** (Supplement 1), S82–S84.

Lawler, J. (1991) *Behind the Screens: Nursing, Somology and the Problem of the Body*. Melbourne: Churchill Livingstone.

Lee, D. (2002) The psychological management of rape and PTSD: clinical issues, assessment and treatment. In: Miller, D., Green, J. (eds) *The Psychology of Sexual Health*. Oxford: Blackwell Science.

Lewis, S., Bor, R. (1994) Nurses' knowledge of and attitudes towards sexuality and the relationship of these with nursing practice. *Journal of Advanced Nursing* **20**, 251–259.

Lupton, D., McCarthy, S., Chapman, S. (1995a) 'Doing the right thing': the symbolic meanings and experiences of having an HIV antibody test. *Social Science and Medicine* **41**, 2, 173–180.

Lupton, D., McCarthy, S., Chapman, S. (1995b) 'Panic bodies': discourses on risk and HIV antibody testing. *Sociology of Health and Illness* **17**, 1, 89–108.

Lynch, P.G. (1988) Psychiatric, legal and moral issues of herpes simplex infection. *Journal of the American Academy of Dermatology* **18**, 173–176.

MacFarlane, L. (1998) *Diagnosis: Homophobic: The Experiences of Lesbians, Gay Men and Bisexuals in Mental Health Services.* London: PACE.

Maguire, P. Parkes, C.M. (1998) Surgery and loss of body parts. In: Parkes, C.M., Markus, A. (eds) *Coping with Loss.* London: BMJ Books.

Mason, A., Palmer, A. (1996) *Queerbashing: A National Survey of Hate Crimes against Lesbians and Gay Men.* London: Stonewall.

Masters, W.H., Johnson, V.E. (1966) *Human Sexual Response.* London: Churchill.

Masters, W. H., Johnson, V.E. (1970) *Human Sexual Inadequacy.* London: Churchill.

Masters, W.H., Johnson, V.E. (1976) Principles of the new sex therapy. *American Journal of Psychiatry* **133**, 548–554.

Mathers, N., Bramley, M., Draper, K., Snead, S., Tobert, A. (1994) Assessment of training in psychosexual medicine. *British Medical Journal* **308**, 969–972.

Matocha, L., Waterhouse, J.K. (1993) Current nursing practice related to sexuality. *Research in Nursing and Health* **16**, 371–378.

Matthews, P. (1998) Sexual history taking in primary care. In: Carter, Y., Moss, C., Weyman, A. (eds) *RCGP Handbook of Sexual Health in Primary Care.* London: Royal College of General Practitioners.

Maughan, K., Clarke, C. (2001) The effect of a clinical nurse specialist in gynaecological oncology on quality of life and sexuality. *Journal of Clinical Nursing* **10**, 221–229.

Maw, R.D., Reitano, M., Roy, M. (1998) An international survey of patients with genital warts: perceptions regarding treatment and impact on lifestyle. *International Journal of STD & AIDS* **9**, 571–578.

McCarthy, B.W. (1990) Treating sexual dysfunction associated with prior sexual trauma. *Journal of Sex and Marital Therapy* **16**, 3, 142–146.

McColl, R. (1994) Homosexuality and mental health services. *British Medical Journal* **308**, 550–551.

McGuire, H., Hawton, K. (2001) Interventions for vaginismus (Cochrane Review). In: The Cochrane Library, Issue 2, 2001. Oxford: Update Software.

McHale, J. (1998) Confidentiality and access to health care records. In: McHale, J., Tingle, J., Peysner, J. (eds) *Law and Nursing.* Oxford: Butterworth–Heinemann.

McNall, A. (2000) Skills for sensitivity. In: Wilson, H., McAndrew, S. (eds) *Sexual Health.* London: Baillière Tindall.

McNally, I., Adams, N. (2000) Psychosexual issues. In: Neal, C., Davies, D. (eds) *Issues in Therapy with Lesbian, Gay, Bisexual and Transgender clients.* Buckingham: Open University Press.

Meerabeau, L. (1999) The management of embarrassment and sexuality in health care. *Journal of Advanced Nursing* **29**, 6, 1507–1513.

Miller, D., Acton, T.M.G., Hedge, B. (1988) The worried well: their identification and management. *Journal of the Royal College of Physicians of London* **22**, 3, 158–165.

Milton, M., Coyle, A. (1999) Lesbian and gay affirmative psychotherapy: issues in theory and practice. *Sexual and Marital Therapy* **14**, 1, 43–59.

Montford, H., Skrine, R. (eds) *Contraceptive Care: Meeting Individual Needs*. London: Chapman & Hall.

Moore, L. (1998) The experience of rape. *Nursing Standard* **12**, 48, 49–56.

Morrisey, M., Rivers, I. (1998) Applying the Mims–Swenson sexual health model to nurse education: offering an alternative focus on sexuality and health care. *Nurse Education Today* **18**, 488–495.

Morse, J.M. (1991) Negotiating commitment and involvment in the nurse–patient relationship. *Journal of Advanced Nursing* **16**, 455–468.

Muir, A. (2000) Counselling patients who have sexual difficulties. *Professional Nurse* **15**, 11, 723–726.

Mullen, P.E., Martin, J.L., Anderson, J.C., Romans, S.E., Herbison, G.P. (1994) The effect of child sexual abuse on social, interpersonal and sexual function in adult life. *British Journal of Psychiatry* **165**, 35–47.

Murphy, M. (1998) The neuroendocrine basis of sexuality and organic dysfunction. In: Freeman, H., Pullen, I. Stein, G., Wilkinson, G. (eds) *Seminars in Psychosexual Disorders*. London: Gaskell.

Nelson, S. (1999) Psychosexual issues in sexual health care. In: Weston, A. (ed.) *Sexually Transmitted Infections*. London: Nursing Times Books.

Nichols, K.A. (1993) *Psychological Care in Physical Illness* (second edition). London: Chapman & Hall.

Nicolson, P. (1998) Talking about sexuality and sexual problems. In: Bayne, R., Nicolson, P., Horton, I. (eds) *Counselling and Communication Skills for Medical and Health Practitioners*. British Psychological Society, Leicester: BPS Books.

Nye, R. (ed.) (1999) *Sexuality*. Oxford: Oxford University Press.

Odets, W. (1995) *In the Shadow of the Epidemic: Being HIV-Negative in the Age of Aids*. London: Cassell.

O'Driscoll, M. (1994) Midwives, childbirth and sexuality 2: men and sex. *British Journal of Midwifery* **2**, 2, 74.

Paff, B.A. (1985) Sexual dysfunction in gay men requesting treatment. *Journal of Sex and Marital Therapy* **11**, 3–18.

Parkes, C.M. (1998) Grief that is overlooked, hidden, or discouraged. In: Parkes, C.M., Markus, A. (eds) *Coping with Loss*. London: BMJ Books.

Parkes, C.M., Markus, A. (eds) (1998) *Coping with Loss*. London: BMJ Books.

Patel, R., Cowan, F.M., Barton, S.E. (1997) Advising patients with genital herpes. *British Medical Journal* **314**, 85–86.

Penman, J. (1998) Action research in the care of patients with sexual anxieties. *Nursing Standard* **13**, 13–15, 47–50.

Petrak, J. (2002) The psychological impact of sexual assault. In: Petrak, J., Hedge, B. (eds) (2002) *The Trauma of Sexual Assault*. Chichester: John Wiley & Sons Ltd.

Petrak, J., Hedge, B. (eds) (2002) *The Trauma of Sexual Assault*. Chichester: John Wiley & Sons Ltd.

Platzer, H., James, T. (2000) Lesbians' experiences of healthcare. *NT Research* **5**, 3, 194–202.

Plaut, S.M. (1997) Boundary violations in professional–client relationships: overview and guidelines for prevention. *Sexual and Marital Therapy* **12**, 1, 77–94.

Pollen, R. (1999) Honest or irresponsible? The reluctant couple therapist. *Institute of Psychosexual Medicine Journal* **21**, 3–7.

Pollen, R. (2001) Cultural aspects of sexual difficulties. *Institute of Psychosexual Medicine Journal* **26**, February, 4–11.

Ralph, D., McNicholas, T. (2000) UK management guidelines for erectile dysfunction. *British Medical Journal* **321**, 499–503.

Ramage, M. (1998) Management of sexual problems. ABC of sexual health. *British Medical Journal* **317**, 1509–1512.

Randall, S. (1998) Intimate examinations. *British Journal of Family Planning* **24**, 83–84.

Raphael-Leff, J. (1991) *Psychological Processes of Childbearing*. London: Chapman & Hall.

Ratigan, B. (1997) Counselling people affected by HIV and AIDS. In Palmer, S., McMahon, G. (eds) *Handbook of Counselling* (second edition). London: Routledge.

RCN (1994) *The Nursing Care of Lesbians and Gay Men: An RCN Statement*. Issues in Nursing and Health 26. London: Royal College of Nursing.

RCN (2000) *Sexuality and Sexual Health in Nursing Practice*. London: Royal College of Nursing.

RCOG (1997) *Intimate Examinations: Report of the Working Party*. London: Royal College of Obstetricians and Gynaecologists Press.

RCOG (1999) Primary and secondary infertility care. *Nursing Standard* **13**, 45, 31.

Read, J. (1999) Sexual problems associated with infertility, pregnancy and ageing. ABC of sexual health. *British Medical Journal* **318**, 587–589.

Riley, A.J., Riley, E.J. (1988) Sex therapy in patients with physical problems. In: Cole, M., Dryden, W. (eds) *Sex Therapy in Britain*. Buckingham: Open University Press.

Robbins, I., Bender, M.P., Finnis, S.J. (1997) Sexual harassment in nursing. *Journal of Advanced Nursing* **25**, 1, 163–169.

Roberts, M. (1993) The method and its meaning. In: Montford, H., Skrine, R. (eds) *Contraceptive Care: Meeting Individual Needs*. London: Chapman & Hall.

Rogers, J.E. (1989) Presentation of a psychosexual problem. In: Skrine, R.L. (ed.) *Introduction to Psychosexual Medicine*. Carlisle: Montana Press.

Rogers, P. (1999) The hidden survivors. *Nursing Standard* **13**, 24, 16–17.

Rosen, R.C., Leiblum, S.R. (1995) Treatment of sexual disorders in the 1990s: an integrated approach. *Journal of Consulting and Clinical Psychology* **63**, 6, 877–890.

Rosser, B.R.S., Short, B.J., Thurmes, P.J., Coleman, E. (1998) Anodyspareunia, the unacknowledged sexual dysfunction: a validation study of painful receptive anal intercourse and its psychosexual concomitants in homosexual men. *Journal of Sex and Marital Therapy* **24**, 281–292.

Rutter, M. (2000a) Section 2: Life span, emotional development and sexuality (chapters 7–12). In: Wells, D. (ed.) *Caring for Sexuality in Health and Illness*. Edinburgh: Churchill Livingstone.

Rutter, M. (2000b) Emotional and Psychosexual Nursing in Impaired Fertility. Caring for Sexuality in Health and Illness. Papers given at the study day on 18 November 2000 organised by the Association of Psychosexual Nursing in Association with the Liverpool Women's Hospital. London: Association of Psychosexual Nursing.

Savage, J. (1987) *Nurses, Gender and Sexuality*. London: Heinemann Nursing.

Savage, J. (1990) Sexuality and nursing care: setting the scene. *Nursing Standard* **4**, 37, 24–25.

Savage, W., Reader, F. (1984) Sexual activity during pregnancy. *Midwife, Health Visitor and Community Nurse* **20**, 398–401.

Schreier, B.A. (1998) Of shoes, and ships, and sealing wax: the faulty and specious assumptions of sexual reorientation therapies. *Journal of Mental Health Counseling* **20**, 4, 305–314.

Scoular, A., Duncan, B., Hart, G. (2001) 'That sort of place ... where filthy men go ...': a qualitative study of women's perceptions of genitourinary medicine services. *Sexually Transmitted Infections* **77**, 340–343.

Segraves, R.T. (1998) Antidepressant-induced sexual dysfunction. *Journal of Clinical Psychiatry* **54** (Supplement 4), 48–54.

Segraves, R.T., Segraves, K.B. (1998) Pharmacotherapy for sexual disorders: advantages and pitfalls. *Sexual and Marital Therapy* **13**, 3, 295–309.

Selby, J. (1989) Psychosexual nursing. In: Skrine, R.L. (ed.) *Introduction to Psychosexual Medicine*. Carlisle: Montana Press.

Selby, J. (2000) Section 3: Coaching for psychosexual awareness (chapters 1318). In: Wells D. (ed.) *Caring for Sexuality in Health and Illness*. Edinburgh: Churchill Livingstone.

Selby, J. (2001) Psychosexual and emotional care. In: Andrews G. (ed.) *Women's Sexual Health* (second edition). London: Baillière Tindall.

Shah, D., Button, J.C. (1998) The relationship between psychological factors and recurrent genital herpes simplex virus. *British Journal of Health Psychology* **3**, 191–213.

Shaw, J.A., Rosenfield, B.L. (1987) Psychological and sexual aspects of genital herpes in women. *Journal of Psychosomatic Obstetrics and Gynecology* **6**, 101–109.

Shelley, C. (ed.) (1998) *Contemporary Perspectives on Psychotherapy and Homosexualities*. London: Free Association Books.

Sherr, L. (1995) Coping with psychosexual problems in the context of HIV infection. *Sexual and Marital Therapy*, **10**, 3, 307-318.

Sherr, L., Green, J. (1996) Dying, bereavement and loss. In: Green, J., McCreaner, A. (eds) *Counselling in HIV Infection and AIDS* (second edition). Oxford: Blackwell Science.

Shires, A., Miller, D. (1998) A preliminary study comparing psychological factors associated with erectile dysfunction in heterosexual and homosexual men. *Sexual and Marital Therapy* **13**, 1, 37–49.

Silman, R. (1995) What is fertility counselling? In: Jennings, S.E. (ed.) *Infertility Counselling*. Oxford: Blackwell Science.

Silverman, D., Perakyla, A. (1990) AIDS counselling: the interactional organization of talk about 'delicate' issues. *Sociology of Health and Illness* **12**, 3, 293–318.

Simon, G. (1996) Working with people in relationships. In: Davies, D., Neal, C. (eds) *Pink Therapy: A Guide for Counsellors and Therapists Working with Lesbian, Gay and Bisexual clients*. Buckingham: Open University Press.

Skrine, R.L. (1989) *Introduction to Psychosexual Medicine*. Carlisle: Montana Press.

Skrine, R., Montford, H. (eds) (2001) Psychosexual Medicine: An Introduction (second edition). London: Arnold.

Smith, A. (1989) The problem is recognised – what next? In: Skrine, R.L. (ed.) *Introduction to Psychsexual Medicine*. Carlisle: Montana Press.

Smith, A. (2001) The skills of psychosexual medicine. In: Skrine, R., Montford, H. (eds) *Psychosexual Medicine: An Introduction* London: Arnold.

Sontag, S. (1991) *Illness as Metaphor and AIDS and Its Metaphors*. London: Penguin Books.

Southern, S. (1999) Facilitating sexual health: intimacy enhancement techniques for sexual dysfunction. *Journal of Mental Health Counseling* **12**, 1, 15–32.

Spence, S. (1991) *Psychosexual Therapy: A Cognitive Behavioural Approach*. London: Chapman & Hall.

Stead, M.L., Fallowfield, L., Brown, J.M., Selby, P. (2001) Communication about sexual problems and sexual concerns in ovarian cancer: qualitative study. *British Medical Journal* **323**, 836–837.

Steele, J., Andrews, G. (2001) Common gynaecological problems. In: Andrews, G. (ed.) *Women's Sexual Health* (second edition). London: Baillière Tindall.

Stravynski, A., Gaudette, G., Lesage, A., Arbel, N., Petit, P., Clerc, D. et al. (1997) The treatment of sexually dysfunctional men without partners: a controlled study of three behavioural group approaches. *British Journal of Psychiatry* **170**, 338–344.

Summerside, J. (1999) *Incorporating HIV Prevention into HIV Treatment Work*. A briefing for treatment information workers, health advisers and clinicians. The Terrence Higgins Trust, London.

Tasker, F., McCann, D. (1999) Affirming patterns of adolescent sexual identity: the challenge. *Journal of Family Therapy* **21**, 30–54.

Taylor, B. (1999) 'Coming out' as a life transition: homosexual identity formation and its implications for health care practice. *Journal of Advanced Nursing* **30**, 2, 520–525.

Taylor, C.A., Keller, M.L., Egan, J.J. (1997) Advice from affected persons about living with human papillomavirus infection, *Image. Journal of Nursing Scholarship* **29**, 1, 27–32.

Taylor, I., Robertson, A. (1994) The health needs of gay men: a discussion of the literature and implications for nursing. *Journal of Advanced Nursing* **20**, 560–566.

Tiefer, L. (1991) Historical, scientific, clinical and feminist criticisms of 'The Human Sexual Response Cycle' model. *Annual Review of Sexual Research* **2**, 1–23.

Tiefer, L. (1994) Three crises facing sexology. *Archives of Sexual Behaviour* **23**, 4, 361–374.

Tomlinson, J. (1998) Taking a sexual history. ABC of sexual health. *British Medical Journal* **317**, 1573–1576.

Trenchard, L., Warren, H. (1984) *Something to Tell You*. London: London Gay Teenage Group.

Trudel, G., Turgeon, L., Piche, L. (2000) Marital and sexual aspects of old age. *Sexual and Relationship Therapy* **15**, 4, 381–406.

Tunnadine, P. (1999) 25 years: the Institute, past, present and future. Once upon a time. *Institute of Psychosexual Medicine Journal* **23**, 2–4.

Turner, R. (1999) Ordinary people. *Nursing Standard* **14**, 1, 22.

UKCC (1992) *Code of Professional Conduct*. London: United Kingdom Central Council for Nursing, Midwifery and Health Visiting.

UKCC (1996a) *Guidelines for Professional Practice*. London: United Kingdom Central Council for Nursing, Midwifery and Health Visiting.

UKCC (1996b) *Position Statement on Clinical Supervision for Nursing and Health Visiting*. London: United Kingdom Central Council for Nursing, Midwifery and Health Visiting.

UKCC (1999) *Practitioner–client Relationships and the Prevention of Abuse*. London: United Kingdom Central Council for Nursing, Midwifery and Health Visiting.

Ussher, JM, Baker, CD. (eds) (1993) *Psychological Perspectives on Sexual Problems*. London: Routledge.

Vanhegan, G. (2001) Problems with female orgasm. In: Skrine, R., Montford, H. (eds) *Psychosexual Medicine: An Introduction* (second edition). London: Arnold.

Von Krogh, G., Lacey, C.J.N., Gross, G., Barrasso, R., Schneider, A. (2000) European course on HPV associated pathology: guidelines for primary physicians for diagnosis and management of anogenital warts. *Sexually Transmitted Infections* **76**, 162–168.

Wakley, G. (1993) Psychosexual problems in the contraceptive consultation. In: Montford, H., Skrine, R. (eds) *Contraceptive Care: Meeting Individual Needs*. London: Chapman & Hall.

Wakley, G. (1998) Sexual problems in primary care. In: Carter, Y., Moss, C., Weyman, A. (eds) *RCGP Handbook of Sexual Health in Primary Care*. London: Royal College of General Practitioners.

Waldby, C. (1996) *AIDS and the Body Politic: Biomedicine and Sexual Difference*. London: Routledge.

Waterhouse, J. (1996) Nursing practice related to sexuality: a review and recommendations. *NT Research* **1**, 6, 412–418.

Watson, J.P., Davies, T. (1997) Psychosexual problems. ABC of mental health. *British Medical Journal* **315**, 239–242.

Webb, C. (1985) *Sexuality, Nursing and Health*. Chichester: John Wiley & Sons.

Webster, C., Heath, H. (2001) Sexuality and people with disability or chronic illness. In: Heath, H., White, I. (eds) *The Challenge of Sexuality in Health Care*. Oxford: Blackwell Science.

Webster, L. (2001) Disorders of sexual preference and gender identity. In: Skrine, R., Montford, H. (eds) *Psychosexual Medicine: An Introduction* (second edition). London: Arnold.

Wells, A. (1997) *Cognitive Therapy of Anxiety Disorders*. Chichester: John Wiley & Sons.

Wells, D. (ed.) (2000) Caring for Sexuality in Health and Illness, Edinburgh: Churchill Livingstone.

White, I. (2001) Facilitating sexual expression: challenges for contemporary practices, In: Health, H., White, I. (eds) *The Challenge of Sexuality in Health Care*. Oxford: Blackwell Science.

Whitmore, J. (2001) Problems with ejaculation. In: Skrine, R., Montford, H. (eds) *Psychosexual Medicine: An Introduction* (second edition). London: Arnold.

WHO (1986) *Concepts for Sexual Health, EUR/ICP/MCH 521P*. Copenhagen: World Health Organization Regional Office for Europe.

WHO (1992) *ICD-10 International Classification of Diseases* (tenth edition). Geneva: World Health Organization.

Willis, E. (1992) The social relations of HIV testing technology. In: Scott, S., Williams, G., Platt, S., Thomas, H. (eds) *Private Risks and Public Dangers, Explorations in Sociology*. No: 43 Aldershot: Avebury.

Wilson, H. (2000) Sex and statutory bodies. In: Wilson, H., McAndrew, S. (eds) *Sexual Health*. London: Baillière Tindall.

Wilson, H., McAndrew, S. (eds) (2000) *Sexual Health*. London: Baillière Tindall.

Wilton, T. (2000) *Sexualities in Health and Social Care*. Buckingham: Open University Press.

Woolley, P. (1997) Psychological responses to a diagnosis of STD. *British Journal of Sexual Medicine* March/April, 6–8.

Wurr, C.J., Partridge, I.M. (1997) The prevalence of a history of childhood sexual abuse in an acute adult inpatient population. *Child Abuse and Neglect* **20**, 9, 867–872.

Wylie, K. (1994) Psychosexual aspects of infertility. *British Journal of Sexual Medicine* **21**, 3, 6–8.

Wylie, K. (1998) Physical treatments for sexual dysfunctions. In: Freeman, H., Pullen, I., Stein, G., Wilkinson, G. (eds) *Seminars in Psychosexual Disorders* London: Gaskell.

Zandvliet, T. (2000) Transgender issues in therapy. In: Neal, C., Davies, D. (eds) *Issues in Therapy with Lesbian, Gay, Bisexual and Transgender Clients*. Buckingham: Open University Press.

Zolese. G., Blacker, C.V.R. (1992) The psychological complications of therapeutic abortion. *British Journal of Psychiatry* **160**, 742–749.

Index

173

Balint, Michael 91
Balint-style psychosexual seminar groups 14,
	47
barbituates 59
Bartholin's cyst 81
Beaumont Society 150
Beaumont Trust 155
behaviour therapy 89
behavioural-systems approach to
	psychosexual therapy 89
beliefs and attitudes about sexual behaviour
	see sexual knowledge and beliefs and
	sexual myths
beneficience 17
benzodiazepines 59
bereavement
	effects on sexual response 4, 81
	hidden losses 68, 100, 105
	loss of a child 105
	loss of a partner 67, 68
	process of bereavement 81
	psychosexual sequelae of
		bereavement 68, 70, 129
	termination of pregnancy 105
betrayal see traumagenic dynamics
bestiality 148
bisexuality 3, 22
blame 101,105,135,137,139
boundaries
	preventing boundary violations 26,
		29, 30, 33, 143, 144
	requirement for the safety of patients
		18
	role in the nurse-patient relationship
		12, 18, 32, 33
breast
	cancer 60, 61, 63
	changes during sexual response 52
	surgery 153
British Association of Sexual and
	Relationship Therapists (BASRT) 94,
	155
British National Formulary 61
buserelin 61

cancer 60,61,63,79
CancerBACUP 156
candidiasis 125
cardiovascular disease 55, 62, 78
catheterization 39
cerebrovascular accident (CVA) 55
cervix

cervical carcinoma 81
cervical smears 14, 39, 134
	requests for a cervical smear as a
		presenting behaviour 35
change of life see menopause
chaperones 30, 40
Child: Infertility Education and Counselling
	156
childbirth
	as a precipitant for sexual problems
		70, 81,104
	distress associated with childbirth
		104, 105, 110
	fears about childbirth 81
	hormonal changes 78
	psychosexual problems following
		childbirth 104
	reactions of partners following
		childbirth 104
	stillbirth 106, 110
childhood sexual abuse (CSA)
	CSA and mental health 138, 141
	definitions of CSA 138
	disclosure of CSA 132, 138, 142, 143
	long term effects of CSA on social,
		interpersonal and sexual
		functioning 9, 81, 141, 143, 145
	responding to disclosures of CSA
		142–145
	traumagenic dynamics of CSA 139,
		140
	see also Abuse
chlamydia 124–126, 136
chronic renal failure 56
cimetidine 61
clinical nurse specialists 60
clinical psychology 94, 143
clinical supervision 26, 8, 30, 33, 47
clitoris
	changes to clitoris during sexual
		response 52, 53, 78
	hypertrophic clitoris 153
Code of Professional Conduct (UKCC) 19,
	20, 21, 26
cognitive behavioural therapy 89, 130, 138
'coming out' 113–115, 153
communication difficulties
	as a cause and manifestation of sexual
		and relationship problems 67, 68,
		71, 73, 90, 105,127, 129